Advance Praise for *Improving Medication Ad*
How to Talk with Patients Al

"In the following pages, you are in for a treat. You are about to enter the very soul of what we do, and you could not find a better guide."

> C. Everett Koop, MD, ScD
> Former Surgeon General of the United States (1981-1989)
> Senior Scholar, C. Everett Koop Institute at Dartmouth

"A bright and refreshing writing style, packed with unusually insightful interviewing tips. Medication issues are central, complex, and controversial in the era of evidence-based medicine and shared decision-making; and Dr. Shea's book is simply the best resource available on communicating with people about their medications."

> Robert E. Drake, MD, PhD
> Andrew Thomson Professor of Psychiatry
> Dartmouth Medical Schools

"Shawn Shea, a rare Lincolnesque physician, wrassles to the ground the tough problem of improving medication adherence. Blissfully short, blessedly succinct - written with gimlet-eyed clarity and eloquence - this book is a boon for any clinician."

> Mack Lipkin, MD
> Founding President of the American Academy on Physician
>   and Patient
> Professor of Medicine
> NYU Medical Center

"A valuable book for even the most experienced clinician from primary care to endocrinology. Dr. Shea brings rich insights to a topic (what words we choose as we introduce medications and address their side-effects), that is seldom discussed in training. He reminds us that our words are as important a part of the pharmacopoeia as the medications themselves."

> John F. Steiner, MD, MPH
> Director of the Colorado Health Outcomes Program
> Professor of Medicine, Preventive Medicine and Biometrics
> University of Colorado

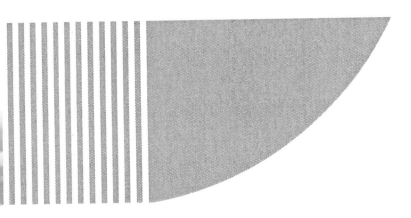

Improving Medication Adherence

How to Talk with Patients About Their Medications

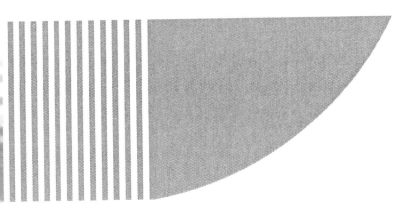

Improving Medication Adherence

How to Talk with Patients About Their Medications

Shawn Christopher Shea, M.D.

Director, Training Institute for
Suicide Assessment and Clinical Interviewing

Adjunct Assistant Professor of Psychiatry,
Dartmouth Medical School

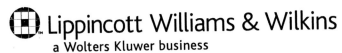 Lippincott Williams & Wilkins

a Wolters Kluwer business

Philadelphia · Baltimore · New York · London
Buenos Aires · Hong Kong · Sydney · Tokyo

Acquisition Editor: Charley Mitchell
Project Manager: Jennifer Jett

Production Services: Maryland Composition Co., Inc.
Printer: R. R. Donnelley & Sons

Library of Congress Cataloging-in-Publication Data

Shea, Shawn C.
  Improving medication adherence: how to talk with patients about their medications / Shawn Christopher Shea.
      p. ; cm.
    Includes bibliographical references and index.
    ISBN 0-7817-9622-9
    1. Physician and patient.   2. Patient compliance.   3. Patient education.
  4. Clinical interviewing.   I. Title.
    [DNLM: 1. Treatment Refusal.   2. Drug Therapy.   3. Interviews – methods.
  4. Physician-Patient Relations.   W 85 S539h 2006]
  R727.3.S54 2006
  610.69'6 – dc22

2006012591

For questions regarding this continuing medical education activity, please contact the Wolters Kluwer Health Office of Continuing Education, 770 Township Line Road, Suite 300, Yardley, PA 19067; by phone: (215) 521-8635; or by fax: (215) 521-8637.

10 9 8 7 6 5

Dedicated to Paul Farmer
whose compassion and mission embody
what it is to be a physician,
and in thanks for his zany humor and the
wonderful laughter
it has brought to Susan and I

ACKNOWLEDGMENTS

I would like to begin by thanking the Department of Psychiatry at the Dartmouth School of Medicine, and its Chairperson, Alan Green, M.D., for supporting my interviewing training programs. A special thanks goes to the Director of Residency Training, Ron Green, M.D. for all of his enthusiasm for my ideas over the years. With Ron's support, at Dartmouth I have found a true haven for training clinicians in the delicate art of interviewing.

As always, I would also like to thank all the Dartmouth faculty who have served as interviewing mentors during the writing of this book - the so-called "Phantom Gate Club." This group includes Christine Barney, M.D., Stephen Cole, Ph.D., and our newest member Graciana Lapetina, M.D. I respect you all greatly, and it has been a privilege to teach the art of interviewing with such great clinicians and teachers.

I would also like to thank all of the participants in my workshops on "Improving Medication Interest" from around the United States and in Canada. I have learned an immense amount from you that has helped me to help my patients. Many of your tips are included in this book, and I hope that I have done justice to your ideas. It is a much better book because of your wisdom.

A true debt of gratitude goes to all of my former patients and clinicians from the Continuous Treatment Team, for I believe I learned more from you about the art of talking about medications than from anybody else. You taught me much, and I still miss our work together.

It is a delightful pleasure to thank my good friend Ed Hamaty for his review of the manuscript and for all of his support over the years. And, of course, a genuine thanks to Bonnie Rossello who has always believed that part of the magic of medications lies in the words that physicians and other clinicians use to sensitively discuss them.

Concerning the production of the book, I would like to thank Charles W. Mitchell, my editor. Charley, I have wanted to work with you for years. It has been worth the wait! Your input has been invaluable. Your patience and sense of humor much appreciated. The book is distinctly better because of you.

I would also like to thank my copy editor, Angie Kilroy, for her work has tightened and improved the text, as well as Pat Mrozek our production manager at Maryland Composition, who was always putting out the fires with grace and elan. And, a genuine thanks to Jennifer Jett, and all of the production team at Lippincott Williams & Wilkins, who have brought the pages of this book to life. And, finally, a hearty thanks goes to Doug Smock whose wonderful talent created the handsome cover for this book.

As I close, I would like to give a special thanks to the former Surgeon General of the United States C. Everett Koop, M.D., ScD for his suggestions on improving the text and for his most gracious Foreword. I believe that you represent the standard by which all clinicians can judge their ability to form a therapeutic alliance and to know what it means to show compassion.

I could not end without giving my deepest thanks to my wife, Susan, who - as with my previous books - edited every single page of this manuscript, and whose sharp eye and splendid sense of composition have greatly improved it.

S.C.S.

CONTENTS

PREFACE

"The purpose of life is to serve and to show compassion and the will to help others. Only then have we ourselves become true human beings."

Albert Schweitzer, MD

This is a small book about a big topic. In fact, an argument could be made, that the problem of medication nonadherence is one of the, if not *the*, major roadblocks to providing effective care in medical practice today. It clearly should be one of the topics most rigorously addressed by all medical, nursing, physician assistant, and clinical pharmacy students during their training. Having intentionally written the book in an informal and conversational style, I hope that these same students will rapidly feel at home with the pages that follow. They are meant to read with the comfortable familiarity of a bedside consult from a colleague one trusts.

My hope is also that veteran clinicians will feel equally at home perusing the following pages, because their years of clinical experience will provide an entirely different – more powerful lens – with which to play with the following ideas. If I've done my job well, as an experienced clinician reads on, he or she will find interviewing techniques and strategies that validate his or her current practice, provide a handful of immediately useful ideas for his or her future practice, and, most importantly, stimulate him or her to find new answers born from their own clinical wisdom.

The techniques in this book are not provided as the "right way" to increase our patients' interest in their medications but merely as suggestions of various ways of tackling these difficult and sometimes vexing problems. The reader is invited to check out the following techniques, adopt the ones that he or she likes, discard the ones that he or she doesn't, and create ever more powerful solutions that resonate with his or her own interviewing styles and the unique needs of his or her patients.

Before I turn the reader loose to follow up on my invitation, I should mention where the interviewing tips, that fill the pages of this book, have originated.

Over the past seven years, as the Director of the Training Institute for Suicide Assessment and Clinical Interviewing (TISA) (information available at http://www.suicideassessment.com), it has been my privilege to present workshops on medication adherence and other aspects of clinical interviewing to primary care physicians, psychiatrists, nurses, clinical pharmacists, and case managers (on teams managing diseases as diverse as CHF and diabetes to schizophrenia) from around the country. At each workshop I ask my workshop participants to stop me if any of the ideas that I suggest seem impractical in a primary care clinic or in a community mental health setting. In the following pages, I share only those ideas that have passed the "acid test" of their discerning judgment.

More importantly, I always invite the participants of my workshops to share the tips that they have found to be most useful in their daily practices – their private cache of clinical pearls. This book is a direct result of these workshops. It is a compilation of the practical tips, suggested at my workshops, coupled with the lessons that I've learned in my own clinical practice over the years.

Concerning my personal ideas for improving medication interest, I should state that they originated far from the world of the ivory tower. For almost five years I directed a frontline "in the trenches" psychiatric team that focused upon the thorny issues surrounding adherence. This team provided outreach to severely impaired psychotic patients at a community mental health center. Our patients were hidden away in the rural back roads and small towns of southern New Hampshire. These teams, known as Continuous Treatment Teams (sometimes called *ACT teams*), were designed to provide care for only the most seriously impaired of mental health patients.

For example, to be eligible for care under our team, the patient had to have either out-of-control schizophrenia or bipolar disorder. In addition, the patient also had to have either active alcohol or street drug abuse. Furthermore, he or she had to have one or several of the following: multiple suicide attempts, multiple acts of violence, or multiple hospitalizations. Needless to say, as these patients first joined our team, they were not big medication advocates. Indeed, our clinical challenge was, in essence, to win the Super Bowl of nonadherence.

Our efforts were monitored by a research study run by Robert Drake, MD, one of the most gifted clinicians with whom I have ever had the pleasure to be associated, and sponsored by the Robert Wood Johnson Foundation. At the end of four years, their monitoring efforts revealed that we were able to decrease the number of hospital days per year of these patients, when compared to other more traditional case-management teams, by twenty days per year. In addition, during this time, there were no suicides with this highly vulnerable group of patients.

Much of our success seemed to be secondary to the strikingly high medication adherence that we were able to achieve with many of our patients. And, I am convinced that it was these same patients that taught us how to do it. We asked and subsequently explored with each of our patients, how we could increase their interest in taking psychotropic agents such as antipsychotics – medications that, I might add, can have some nasty side-effects. The answers that they gave, one way or the other, always seemed to return to the complexities and elusive exchanges of the physician-patient relationship. The answers had to do with how we saw them, how they saw us, and how we, together, saw our alliance against their disease. Their answers, equally true for a person suffering from diabetes as for a person suffering from schizophrenia, provide much of the practical wisdom that follows in this book.

Finally, I should add that for over twenty years, it has been my great pleasure to study and write about the art of interviewing. I have specialized in developing methods for training both inexperienced and experienced clinicians.

Over these years I have become convinced of the necessity of providing the clinician, not only with sound principles, but also with direct examples of how to implement these principles. The clinician needs to see the exact phrases and questions that can transform a sound principle into a sound practice. In the last analysis, mastering interviewing is probably not as dependent upon knowing what to say than upon knowing how, and when, to say it. Thus, as was the case with my previous books, I have tried to pack this primer with sample questions and concrete interviewing strategies.

I should add a brief note about the title of this book. As readers will see, I hope that the terms "medication compliance" and "medication adherence" will some day be replaced with the term "medication interest." If the message of this book hits home, future editions of this book will be entitled "Improving Medication Interest," for the term will be widely recognized. Until that time, I have used the more commonly understood term - adherence - to avoid confusion about the topic of the book.

In closing, I hope the reader enjoys the following pages. I certainly enjoyed writing them. I truly believe that, in the last analysis, it is a privilege to be a physician, a nurse, a physician assistant, a clinical pharmacist, or a case manager.

Our journey, as physicians and healers, is a rich one. In our efforts to provide help to our patients we sometimes succeed and we sometimes fail, but we always learn. As we move more deeply into their pains and their fears, we encounter the reflections of those pains and fears – their hopes and expectations. Our medications become their hope for relief and their expectations are that our medications will provide it. Sometimes they do, sometimes they don't.

It is here, within the chaotic world where suffering and compassion meet and sometimes collide, that we move ever more deeply into the souls of our patients. Once there, we have the great privilege, as Albert Schweitzer observed, to suddenly know what it is "to become true human beings." These moments are the moments that define our livelihoods as physicians, nurses, physician assistants, clinical pharmacists, and case managers. This book is about such moments.

Shawn Christopher Shea, MD

FOREWORD

Let me begin with a bias – a strong one. After four decades of clinical practice and 25 years of monitoring it from the sidelines (eight of them from the best seat in the house as Surgeon General), I have become convinced that the cornerstone of all healing in medicine lies within the mysterious bond that grows between the physician and the patient. Call it what you will – *bond, alliance, relationship* – it is the heart and soul of medicine.

It is one of the reasons that I was so pleased to be the Senior Scholar of the C. Everett Koop Institute created at Dartmouth Medical School, dedicated to understanding these mysteries. It has been my goal to explore these mysteries, to honor those protocols that, by their nature, must remain mysterious and to delineate and teach those processes that can be discerned, made operational, and taught.

I have arrived at a second conclusion – as has the author of this book – a conclusion that is so obvious that it is often not recognized as critical to discuss or even to mention. No medication works inside a bottle. Period. Now let me bridge the relationship between my two conclusions.

Our patients reach for their pill bottles, unscrew their caps, and reap the benefits of our medications almost purely because of the power of their bond with us. They either trust us or they don't. They either feel they have been well informed or they don't. They either feel we care or we don't. All of these patient opinions are the reflection of the ongoing nuances of the physician-patient relationship as it defines itself.

Unfortunately, far too little time is spent in our medical school education, our residency training, and in our ongoing continuing medical education on this most practical of all interviewing skills: talking with patients about their medications. When time is spent on these topics, it is often, in my opinion, wasted with clichés and admonitions to "be empathic" and to build "collaborative relationships." Such goals are laudable, but what is needed is a probing, tenacious attempt to uncover the specific interviewing techniques, choices of words, strategies, nuances, and experiences that talented clinicians use to convey empathy and to build these relationships, not just talk about the need to do so.

I know of no book that has ever addressed this critical set of interviewing skills regarding the specific task of how we talk with our patients about their medications. By necessity, I leaned heavily on my own experience when I led the program, *Take Time To Talk*, giving tips to patient and physician alike about talking to each other; I let each group see and hear what I said to the other.

You are holding in your hands the first book, as far as I know, in the history of medicine, that admonishes physicians to take the time to talk with patients about their medications. It does so with remarkable readability, practicality, and elegance. Reading this book never feels like one is reading a textbook of medicine. Instead, one feels that one is talking informally with a trusted mentor while doing bedside rounds – a mentor who believes in the mission, understands the complexities of the work, and genuinely both enjoys and loves his patients.

Hopefully, Shea's philosophy of enhancing "medication interest," as opposed to enforcing "medication compliance," will become second nature to generations of future medical and nursing students, as well as residents from primary care to psychiatry. I believe his book will become standard reading in all medical and nursing classes on medical interviewing or the physician-patient relationship, because it covers a critical topic in medical interviewing often overlooked – how to talk with patients about their medications.

Improving Medication Adherence is filled with a remarkable number – around forty – specific interviewing techniques and strategies for talking to patients about their medications and their side effects, in a collaborative fashion in the primary care setting, psychiatry, and elsewhere. The principles are equally relevant for talking with our patients about antihypertensives, oral hypoglycemic agents, and antidepressants.

Curiously, the book has come not from a family practitioner or internist but from a psychiatrist, who, in my opinion, did two wise things: (1) He brought the keen observations and principles that are useful in discussing psychiatric agents – notoriously difficult to get patients interested in taking – to the discussion table, and (2) he has distilled his interaction with thousands of primary care clinicians across the country in over 150 workshops, culling from them their very best interviewing techniques concerning all classes of medications, techniques that have proven themselves in the hectic confines of contemporary primary care clinics. Thus, this book, in essence, is written by a psychiatrist but contains the input of hundreds of primary care clinicians, who know what works and what does not work in actual practice no matter what class of medication is being discussed.

I also like the no-nonsense attitude that Shea takes, when he emphasizes that the techniques he describes are not offered as the right way to interview (as if there was a cookbook manner for talking to patients correctly about medications). Instead, he describes them as reasonable ways. He hopes that the reader picks and chooses those techniques that appeal to each specific clinician, for we are all different and must develop our own styles.

Shea also achieves what I view as an even more remarkable goal. He not only engenders in the reader a genuine excitement about interviewing, he also provides a foundation in the principles that are necessary for creating new and effective interviewing strategies. From these principles, the clinician can develop his or her own unique techniques, throughout the ensuing years of his or her career, long after he or she has put the book down. Shea invites the reader to become an innovator, and he gives the reader the necessary tools to be one.

Long ago I learned the power of interviewing technique to enhance my relationships with my patients. For years I had been taught to always address the parents of my patients (I was a pediatric surgeon) by their last names and to be addressed vice versa. So I did. Pediatrics, as opposed to pediatric surgery, is much more homey and first names are "in."

So as the years progressed, I began to realize that when talking with people about life and death decisions about their children or other loved ones, our relationship was not some pseudo-professional exchange of ideas, but an intimate discussion, the closest bond you can have, between people who were building a unique relationship while collaboratively battling frightening diseases and scary surgical procedures, so last names often didn't cut it.

Consequently, when I first introduced myself to a parent or patient, I always addressed them by their last names. But then, I did something special; I gave them control of how I should address them. I simply asked, "Mrs. Jones, how would you like me to address you, by your last name, your first name, or whatever you like?" With this simple question the bond between the healer and those seeking his or her help began.

By the way, if the patient's parents told me they preferred his or her first name, I was not averse to being called by my first name as well – I've been called a lot worse! Also, if the patient insists on being addressed formally by their last name, I simply reciprocate, "It's probably best to call me Dr. Koop."

Over the years I have found that patients enjoy this collaborative work on an important relationship issue – how we want to be addressed – that opens the door to the recognition that we are entering a most special alliance, one where we will be discussing the most intimate of details, sometimes talking about frightening news, such as the presence of cancer or the approach of death, and brainstorming on options, and realizing, together, that sometimes there are no further options. Such are the moments when it is powerful and reassuring to use first names and to even shed a tear or two. In the last analysis, healing is about being human, learning how to allow our science to be guided by our compassion.

In the following pages, you are in for a treat. You are about to enter the very soul of what we do, and you could not find a better guide. With sophistication, wit, astute clinical observation, and a vibrant sense of compassion, Shea throws a brilliant new light on one of the most crucial topics in medicine – improving medication adherence. Packed with practical interviewing techniques and no-nonsense strategies, this little book, in my opinion, is destined to fill a giant void in the training of all medical and nursing students, as well as becoming a classic read for experienced clinicians in search of the art of medicine. My advice is simple – read it.

C. Everett Koop, MD, ScD
Former Surgeon General of the United States (1981–1989)
Senior Scholar, C. Everett Koop Institute at Dartmouth
Elizabeth DeCamp McInerny Professor of Surgery

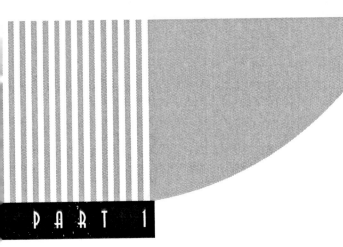

PART 1

When
Patients
Don't
Take
Medications:
Core
Principles

Nonadherence: The Extent of the Problem

"We prescribing clinicians continue to struggle with the most basic of problems: how to get our patients to take the pills that we think they need in the way we think they should. As efficacious as the medications are in research reports and clinical studies, they cannot be effective without moving from the prescription vial to the patient's body."

James M. Ellison, MD, MPH[1]

L ooking back at medical school days, just about every physician can remember a favorite attending sharing some sage advice that went along these lines, "The number one cause of treatment failure is not wrong diagnosis, not wrong drug choice, but poor adherence." As far as clinical axioms go, this one is surprisingly valid.

Over the years, numerous studies have found that patients with chronic diseases take their medications as prescribed only about 50% to 60% of the time.[2] The actual number depends upon the disease in question, but more careful study reveals that about one third of patients comply reasonably well with recommended treatment, about one third have moderate problems with adherence, and about one third take the medicines poorly or not at all.[3] Whether adhering or not, about one third of patients with chronic illnesses have strong reservations about the medications they are on – future examples of discontinuance just waiting to happen.[4]

Statistics aside, many of us don't need to look much further than the nearest mirror to see the ubiquitous nature of nonadherence; I, for one, know that I have not always taken medications exactly the way I was supposed to take them – and I am not alone. Nonadherence is not the sole province of any one type of person. From child to grandparent, from high-school dropout to Rhodes scholar, from a struggling parent in a welfare line in downtown Detroit to an e-business hotshot in a ticket line on Broadway, all types and shapes of people are guilty of "playing" with their meds. Nonadherence is everywhere, it would seem.

Not only is nonadherence not specific to any single type of person, it is not specific to any single type of disease. The list of diseases in which nonadherence has been tagged as particularly commonplace – diabetes, hypertension, hyperlipidemia, heart failure, epilepsy, AIDS, depression, and schizophrenia, to name only a few – reads like a veritable "who's who" of crippling diseases.

Closer review of the literature highlights the havoc that nonadherence (or *noncompliance* as it is still sometimes called) can play in the treatment of specific disease states, such as congestive heart failure (CHF), epilepsy, and depression. The authors of one study of more than 7,000 elderly patients who needed daily digoxin found that they refilled their prescriptions enough times to take their medications for only 111 days of the year – 30% of the time![5] One shudders at picturing these patients abruptly stopping, then starting, then stopping their medications. Easily imaginable are patients madly doubling or tripling any specific dosage when they realize that they have missed some doses and feel a need to catch up. Not the best way to take digoxin.

Another set of researchers found that their epileptic patients managed to take only 76% of their prescribed doses of anti-epileptic drugs, with a range of 3% to 100% adherence.[6] In a study by Katon and colleagues, it was found that a whopping 60% of primary care patients discontinued their antidepressants before completing the recommended 6 months of therapy.[7]

Putting research aside, any clinician who has been in the clinical trenches for even a few years can attest to any medical or nursing student that nonadherence is not a manufactured problem, and it is, in the parlance of contemporary slang, "the real thing." As noted in the Preface, learning the sophisticated interviewing techniques for transforming nonadherence, such as the ones described in this book is, arguably, one of the most important tasks for any student of medicine, nursing, or pharmacy to undertake. Mastering these techniques and creating new ones are, arguably, two of the most important tasks for any veteran clinician to continue throughout the years, for, as we veteran clinicians know all too well, each patient brings us new challenges and, sometimes, in a refreshing light, new lessons. Let us pause for a moment to see where we are.

Clearly, nonadherence is common and is associated with treatment failure, but is it harmful? Do people who fail to take their medications actually become iller? This is a legitimate question, not just a semantic tease, because not all associated phenomena are causal in relation, as we all remember from our undergraduate courses in statistics. Let us see what the data suggest on this point.

In the Beta-Blocker Heart Attack Trial of 1990 (a study of postinfarction treatment approaches) an important finding was discovered among the 2,175 patients who were available for a medication adherence analysis. Those patients who took less than 75% of their medications (as measured in pill counts) had a 2.5-fold increase in mortality compared to those patients who took their medications more assiduously.[8] Now *that's* a finding that will make one reach for the pill bottle more regularly. But it is far from alone.

Data from a study looking at the benefits related to antibiotic adherence show similarly convincing results. For example, a randomized trial of oral antibiotic prophylaxis in patients with cancer showed the following results. Patients who showed good adherence developed fever and infection in only 18% of the cases, contrasted with the development of fever and infection in 54% of those patients with poor adherence.[9]

As one would expect, the field of psychiatry is replete with evidence of the critical role that medication adherence plays in morbidity and mortality in such serious diseases as schizophrenia and bipolar disorder. Sometimes, in looking at outcomes such as suicide, growing evidence shows that mortality rates among nonadherent patients with bipolar disorder are much higher than among adherent patients.[10,11] With our own work, in which we used aggressive home outreach to patients suffering from severe schizophrenia and alcoholism, we were able to decrease hospital days, compared to controls, by 20 days per year per patient. As I stated in the Preface, I am convinced that our success was related to remarkably high medication adherence rates.

It appears evident that adherence helps. But can it be improved through the use of specific physician questions and statements – the focus of our book? I'm convinced, from years of training professionals, that it can be improved substantially. But there is also mounting research evidence to support this case.

Let us look at antidepressant adherence, because antidepressants are one of the most commonly prescribed of medications in both primary care and psychiatric settings – indeed, primary care physicians prescribe more antidepressants than all psychiatrists combined. For example, a fascinating study once again from Katon and colleagues, and spear-headed by Elizabeth Lin of the Group Health Cooperative of Puget Sound, focused upon the early adherence rates of primary care patients. I can't convey their results any more concisely than they did in the synopsis of their article, so it is best to let them speak for themselves:

Approximately 28% of patients stopped taking antidepressants during the first month of therapy, and 44% had stopped taking them by the third month of therapy. Patients who received the following five specific educational messages – 1) take the medication daily; 2) antidepressants must be taken for 2 to 4 weeks for a noticeable effect; 3) continue to take medicine even if feeling better; 4) do not stop taking antidepressant without checking with the physician; and 5) specific instructions regarding what to do to resolve questions regarding antidepressants – were more likely to comply during the first month of antidepressant therapy. Asking about prior experience with antidepressants and discussions about scheduling pleasant activities also were related to early adherence.[12]

The results of the Puget Sound group are highly encouraging, because, in this case, they indicate that specific interviewing statements made during the medication education phase of the appointment can significantly improve adherence.

As the previous study illustrates, not only can specific techniques help to improve adherence, but also there appear to be a lot of them. Each research paper seems to have a slightly different slant. I am consistently surprised at the variety of new ideas that workshop participants provide wherever I go. It seems that within every workshop I give, I hear from the audience a new idea on how to improve adherence. I am convinced that as many new potential ideas on interviewing techniques for improving adherence exist, as there are interviewers and the unique patients whom they are interviewing.

Let me demonstrate how we will fashion a research finding or a specific workshop participant suggestion into a concrete tip in the following pages. In this case, we will look at a research finding that had an impact on my clinical practice the very next day after reading about it. In an ingenious study, Joyce Kramer and colleagues monitored the adherence of patients taking anti-epileptic drugs by having the patients use MEMS bottles.[13] MEMS bottles contain a microprocessor in their caps that record each opening as a presumptive dose, listing the date and time for later retrieval on a microcomputer. Pretty nifty.

The results were surprising. The patients were monitored during all of the days between two consecutive clinic visits at least two months apart. At each visit, serum blood levels were drawn exactly as they would have been in clinical practice. Not only did adherence drop over time with many patients, but also patients fluctuated on how they took their medications over the course of the two months. The 20 patients averaged 88% adherence in the days directly before the first visit to be monitored and 86% adherence in the days directly after the visit. But their adherence dropped to 67% 1 month later. One interesting possibility is that patient adherence may tend to improve with more frequent visits – 2 months being too long in this cohort – as logic would suggest. But there was an even more intriguing finding.

One of the patients showed a problematic pattern of missing more of his medications as the 2 months progressed, but then in the final days before his next scheduled appointment, he took the medications exactly as prescribed. More importantly, by taking the medications correctly, in the 4 days immediately before his next office visit, he managed to get the blood level of his carbamazepine into the mid-range, almost exactly where it had been at his last visit. Now let us see how we can translate this research finding into a practical clinical tip.

PROTOTYPIC TIP #1   Serum blood levels, whether for digoxin, Tegretol, or lithium, are often valued as reliable reflections of medication adherence. But with some patients, especially patients with far spaced appointments, they may convey a false illusion of actual medication adherence. It is very easy to forget meds or to "just not be bothered with them" on certain days. An otherwise conscientious patient who is missing doses rather regularly may return to full medication adherence in the days immediately before an appointment. It would be quite natural to do this because many patients want to appear that they are doing "what is right." Wanting to be viewed by one's doctor as being a reliable patient who "follows doctor's orders" is normal. The subsequent blood level drawn may fall well within acceptable thera- peutic range, thus providing the false appearance of good ongoing adherence. It is useful to complement blood levels with direct questions about adherence between visits even if a patient is showing excellent blood levels.

As we share more and more tips in the following pages, I don't think that we will be disappointed by the intensity of our focus upon the topic of medication adherence. Precious little time for reading exists in our busy worlds, but this is one topic where our time will be well spent, because the problem of medication adherence is going to get worse before it gets better in the years to come. Nonadherence issues will become progressively more time-consuming in all future clinical practices. A simple demographic – the age of our patient population – tells us this is so.

Pressing as the topic of medication adherence is with our typi- cal patient population, it is even more pressing in our care of the older patient. Medication problems take on a new light when the patient is over age 65, as Assumpta Ryan points out in her excel- lent review article on medication adherence issues in older peo- ple, first appearing in the *International Journal of Nursing Studies*.[14] Three key situations complicate the picture with older patients.

First, the physiologic aging process affects absorption, dis- tribution, metabolism, and excretion of medications. The net result is often a narrowing of the therapeutic window with this population. Consequently, smaller errors in adherence can result in bigger problems in care. Inadvertent surges into toxic ranges or precipitous drops out of therapeutic windows can prove to be more frequent outcomes from rather modest problems with nonadherence in this age group.

The second confounding factor with a more aged population is the increased frequency of comorbidity. Many of our elderly patients not only have an additional disorder to their primary problem, but also they frequently have three, four, five, or more disorders. Multisystem disease is so prevalent in this population that the idea of a primary disorder becomes somewhat muted, because such patients frequently have multiple diseases that could kill them if they are not adequately controlled.

Multisystem disorder means multisystem medication regimens. The result is sometimes confusing, not only to the prescribing clinician, but also to the patient's own body. More medications mean more possible drug-drug interactions. We begin to run a fine line as to how much medicine will interact safely with its fellow residents in the bloodstream and how much is problematic. Once again, medication errors – in this case, the patient taking too much – can prove costly.

Our third confounding factor in this age group is that the use of multiple medications can also prove to be quite confusing, in a psychological sense, to the aging patient. For instance, with failing eyesight, bottle labels become harder to read. Problems with concentration and memory may create ever more treacherous adherence pitfalls, heightened by the fact that the older patient may frequently live alone.

With a heightened awareness of the increased ramifications of medication nonadherence in our aging patients, we can bring this introductory chapter to a close. The goal of the chapter was to highlight, in a very real sense, the extent of the nonadherence problem, while hinting that there are a number of potential methods for frequently transforming it.

In the last analysis, the problem of patient nonadherence goes to the very core of our efforts to develop a sound and enduring relationship with our patients. How we resolve the delicate arabesque we call nonadherence is, in many respects, the microcosm to the macrocosm of how we forge our ongoing physician-patient relationship.

Each physician-patient relationship is unique, and each physician-patient relationship must define its own unique set of expectations and methods of joint problem solving. It is often over the issue of "meds" that this definition evolves. The remainder of this book is an effort to show some of the concrete interviewing techniques that can help clinicians from all disciplines to more effectively do their part in defining this potentially powerful alliance – the alliance that helps us to heal when healing is possible and to comfort when it is not.

REFERENCES

1. Ellison JM. Enhancing adherence in the pharmacotherapy treatment relationship. In: Tasman A, Riba M, Silk K, eds. *The Doctor-Patient Relationship in Pharmacotherapy*. New York: Guilford Press; 2000:72.
2. Sackett DL, Snow JC. The magnitude of adherence and nonadherence. In: Haynes R, Sackett D, Taylor D, eds. *Adherence in Health Care*. Baltimore: Johns Hopkins University Press; 1979:11–22.
3. Fedder DO. Managing medication and adherence: physician-pharmacist-patient interaction. *J Am Geriatr Soc* 1982;30:113–117.
4. Practice research a potent force for change, says President. *Pharm J* May 30, 1998;260:791–794.
5. Monane M, Bohn RL, Gurwitz JH, et al. Nonadherence with congestive heart failure therapy in the elderly. *Arch Intern Med* 1994;153:433–437.
6. Cramer JA, Mattson RH, Prevey ML, et al. How often is medication taken as prescribed? A novel assessment technique. *JAMA* 1989;261:3273–3277.
7. Katon W, Von Korff M, Lin E, et al. Adequacy and duration of antidepressant treatment in primary care. *Med Care* 1992;30:67.
8. Horwitz RI, Viscoli CM, Berkman L. Treatment adherence and risk of death after a myocardial infarction. *Lancet* 1990;336:542–545.
9. Pizzo PA, Robichaud KJ, Edwards BK, et al. Oral antibiotic prophylaxis in patients with cancer: a double-blind randomized placebo-controlled trial. *J Pediatr* 1983;102:125–133.
10. Coppen A, Standish-Barry H, Bailey J, et al. Does lithium reduce the mortality of recurrent mood disorders? *J Affect Disord* 1991;23:1–7.
11. Isometsa E, Henriksson M, Lonqvist J. Completed suicide and recent lithium treatment. *J Affect Disord* 1992;26:101–104.
12. Lin EH, Von Korff M, Katon W, et al. The role of the primary care physician in patients' adherence to antidepressant therapy. *Med Care* 1995;33(1):67–74.
13. Cramer JA, Scheyer RD, Mattson RH. Adherence declines between clinic visits. *Arch Intern Med* 1990;150:1509–1510.
14. Ryan AA. Medication adherence and older people: a review of the literature. *Int J Nurs Stud* 1999;36:153–162.

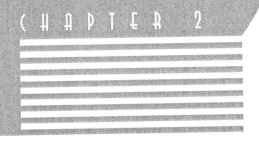

The Crux of the Problem: The Nature of Medication Nonadherence

"The doctor-patient relationship can be restored. But it will take commitment by people on both sides of the stethoscope."[1]

C. Everett Koop, MD

Former U.S. Surgeon General

WHAT IS RESISTANCE? THE TRUTH NO ONE TOLD US ABOUT IN MEDICAL SCHOOL

Medication nonadherence has many roots. Some patients miss medications because of specific cognitive problems. Such problems can range from those of a severe nature – dementia – to the not so severe – everyday forgetfulness. Other patients inappropriately take medications because of confusion over the directions or intellectual limitations on their abilities to follow them. Still, others stop medications because of external limitations – not enough money or no means of transportation to the pharmacy.

A fairly large percentage of patients do not take their medications because they do not want to take them. In short, these patients *choose* not to take the medications that we recommend, or, if they do take them, they choose to take them differently than we prescribe them. We will focus our attention on this latter group of patients in the following pages, because such patients frequent our offices daily, and, unlike the previously mentioned patients, these patients often seem to present insurmountable obstacles.

We can often arrange a ride to the pharmacy for patients requiring transportation and frequently procure sample medications from pharmaceutical companies for patients needing money. Also, we can arrange for family members to distribute medications or provide compartmentalized pill cases to patients coping with memory problems. But we cannot make a patient take a medication that he or she does not want to take. No easy ways exist to transform such personal resistances to taking medications. Or are there?

Our goal in this chapter, and in this book, is to develop a no-nonsense theory as to what causes this type of medication nonadherence, the type characterized by patient choice. But such a theory will be of no value unless it helps us to transform this type of medication nonadherence in our everyday clinical practices. Consequently, our second goal is to use this theory to generate specific statements, questions, and interviewing strategies that can be immediately practiced by us, by our staffs, and by those young clinicians whom we teach.

To understand why our patients choose to not do what we ask – that is, take the medicines that we think can help them – it may be useful to look at why any human being does not do what another human being asks. This question brings us face to face with the provocative topic of "resistance," of which medication nonadherence is but one example, because our patients may also be resistant to dieting, exercising, or stopping smoking. If we can understand how resistance begins, and, even more importantly, how resistance unfolds, intensifies, and sometimes resolves, we may uncover our first hints as to how to transform medication nonadherence and other such clinical gremlins.

A curious, but, ultimately, very useful place to begin our exploration is through a bit of imaginative play. Picture for a moment that we have hired a field anthropologist to help us study and define the nature of "medication noncompliance." Further imagine that we have plopped this anthropologist into one of our primary care offices or psychiatric clinics, on a typically hectic day, to watch us interact with those patients who are either refusing medications or not taking them as prescribed.

As clinicians we know exactly how resistance feels, and if we are really honest with ourselves, most definitions of resistance come down to something rather simple: Resistance occurs when the patient does not do what I want. In some instances, the patient might not take the medications that I suggest. In other instances, he or she may not stop smoking as I suggest. But the bottom line is that the patient is not doing what I want.

At such moments, it is easy for physicians to become appropriately frustrated because we genuinely care about our patients, and we genuinely feel that our medications can help them – sometimes even save their lives. The question now becomes, would our anthropologist agree with our definition of resistance, which we based upon how it feels when we encounter it?

I believe that the answer is likely to be both "yes" and "no." "Yes," in the sense that the definition is correct as far as it goes, and "no," in the sense that it is does not go far enough.

Let us return to our hypothetical anthropologist. We will tell our anthropologist almost nothing about the roles of the two people. We will merely state that, in our culture, what is about to occur between the physician and the patient is called "resistance," and that we would benefit from a scientific description of exactly what is occurring. We will also ask the anthropologist to watch many different clinician-patient examples of resistance, especially examples of medication nonadherence.

After observing hundreds of resistant patient interactions, I believe that our anthropologist would walk out and begin his or her definition of resistance with exactly the same words that we used: "Resistance occurs when the patient does not do what the physician wants." But I believe that our anthropologist would add "and it occurs when the physician does not do what the patient wants." This last caveat is not merely a semantic distinction. It is a profound fact of human nature.

It suggests that in many instances, but not all, when our anthropologist found a physician growing frustrated with a "resistant" patient who did not "get it," there was an equally frustrated patient wondering, "Why doesn't Dr. Shea get it? I don't want to take this drug. It makes me feel bad, and I don't really like taking medications anyway."

From an anthropological perspective, resistance, and more germane to our topic, medication nonadherence is often a two-way street. Resistance is not so much a behavior that one person does, as it is an experience that two people share, with both parties experiencing an unpleasant sensation. Indeed, some patients eventually decide not to come back to a "resistant" physician whom they perceive as always lecturing them to do something that they have no intention of doing, whether it be dieting, exercising, or taking a medication.

I believe that this distinction is the truth that Paul Farmer, the noted physician and anthropologist based in Haiti, meant in a *New Yorker* magazine interview, when he provocatively quipped, "Patients are not noncompliant. Physicians are."[2] You see, that is exactly how patients often see the problem. They think we are the problem, and that we are noncompliant with their views. We think they are the problem, and that they are noncompliant with our views. The anthropologist thinks that we both are the problem; it is the anthropologist who may be closest to the truth.

BOTH SIDES OF THE STETHOSCOPE: HOW RESISTANCE LIVES AND DIES

With a clearer picture of what resistance is, let us explore more thoroughly how it prospers. Common sense tells us that the more intensely one side of a resistant dyad tries to "push" its ideas onto the other side, the more likely the other side will resist those ideas and "push" back. Generally speaking, the more that one perceives being opposed, the more one opposes.

Common sense also tells us that gentle resistances (mild differences of opinion) and not-so-gentle resistances (intense arguments) have one thing in common. For the resistance to resolve, nine times out of ten, one of the people involved must yield, if even just a bit. As one side yields, the other person feels less opposition and, consequently, that person throws back less oppositional intensity.

Naturally, this decrease in oppositional intensity leads the other person, now also perceiving less pressure, to throw even less pressure at the other side and so on. The bottom line is that a gentle see-sawing of de-escalation unfolds.

When one side has the courage to yield, compromise is given birth, whether in a family dispute or at a negotiating table. But what about over an examining table, where both a frustrated physician and a frustrated patient are at loggerheads over the use of a specific medication?

Traditionally, in the fields of medicine and psychotherapy, such clinical resistance was viewed, not as we have described it in this chapter as a joint venture, but as a problem that the patient *has*. Consequently, the techniques for resolving resistance focused upon how to change the patient's supposedly oppositional thoughts, because if one could change the patient's oppositional thinking, then that person might change how the patient behaves. The goal was to break through the patient's resistance and to make the noncompliant patient compliant.

Unfortunately, this traditional model is misleading, because we have seen that resistance is a clashing of two world views – not necessarily a problem with just one world, one end of the stethoscope as C. Everett Koop so cogently began our chapter. Like the proverbial "one hand clapping" one person resisting does not exist. The crux of the matter is simple: If I can lessen how much a patient feels that I am pressuring him or her to take a medication, the likelihood that the patient will choose to take the medication may, paradoxically, increase.

In this regard, perhaps the best way to motivate patients to take medications lies less on focusing on how to change their beliefs and more on focusing how I express my own. I have direct and immediate control over my personal method of expressing my opinions, which means that I will always have something tangible that I can do (i.e., change the wording of my message) whenever a patient is resistant to taking medications. No end exists to the creative solutions that I can bring to the problem, because I can always change my own opinions or the fashion in which I express them. The rest of this book is about the refreshing promise of this one simple idea.

In a practical sense it all comes down to the following principle. Rather than creating the sensation that we are moving "against them," we want our patients to feel that we are moving "with them" – that we are a team, not opposing armies. As we have established so far, this oppositional feeling is often the crux of their resistance and subsequent medication nonadherence.

But how do we avoid this oppositional feeling in clinical practice, if, in truth, the patient actually opposes our beliefs? What do we do if the patient does not want to take his or her medications, to stop smoking, or to start dieting? Must we not be in opposition at such times?

Part of the solution lies in something that we mentioned earlier. What drives the intensity of our patients' resistance is not so much that we are truly opposing them or pressuring them, but that their *perception* is that we are. It is our patients' perceptions of our attitudes that determine whether or not they feel comfortable with our recommendations, not necessarily the reality of the situation.

This patient perception is not created so much by what we say but how we say it. We can hold opposing views from our patient without being an opponent, depending upon the words we choose to share those views. Our words convey not only meaning. They convey relationship.

Let us now see whether our theory can lead us to some practical interviewing techniques that can transform medication nonadherence in everyday practice. To do so we must first develop a more sophisticated understanding of how patients actually decide whether or not to try a medication and to stay on it. Now is the time to look at the stethoscope from the patient's end.

REFERENCES

1. Gordon T, Edwards WS. *Making the Patient Your Partner: Communication Skills for Doctors and Other Caregivers.* Westport, CT: Auburn House; 1997:1.
2. Kidder T. The good doctor. *The New Yorker,* July 10, 2000:40–57.

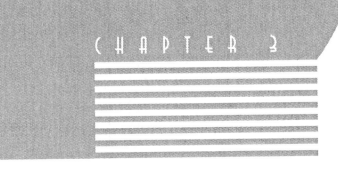

How Do Patients Choose to Take a Medication?

"To desire to take medicine is perhaps the greatest feature which distinguishes man from animals."[1]

Sir William Osler, MD

Renowned Physician (1849–1919)

"I firmly believe that if the whole materia medica as now used could be sunk to the bottom of the sea, it would be all the better for mankind – and all the worse for the fishes."[2]

Oliver Wendell Holmes, Sr.

Renowned Physician (1809–1894)

THE "GREAT DEBATE" IN THEORY

Inside each patient contemplating taking a medication or deciding to stay on it, a debate is waged. For patients who feel most comfortable passively accepting the recommendations of their doctor, it is a relatively quiet matter, without much ado. For patients, who feel more comfortable aggressively evaluating their physician's recommendations, it can be a rather raucous affair, sometimes with much ado about everything. Most patients have a healthy admixture of both perspectives, which enhances their likelihood of being well-informed consumers. But the process of choosing to put a foreign substance into one's body is always a complex one.

The process is as if there were dueling lawyers inside the courtroom of each patient's mind. One lawyer sees only the very real benefits of medications and taps into the deep leanings of the human spirit for almost magical relief, as Sir William Osler describes in the opening epigram of the chapter. The other sees only the very real dangers of medications and taps into the equally deep doubts of the human psyche, as Oliver Wendell Holmes, Sr., so acerbically attests. Across this wide spectrum, the bottom line remains the same for all patients, that is, ultimately, they have to make a choice.

It is not an easy choice. The data are sometimes conflicting. Determining whether the advice of the physician is biased or unbiased can be difficult. To return to our courtroom analogy, is this expert witness a "hired gun" or a "stalwart advocate" for truth? How is a patient to know for sure? Understanding how patients make this decision is at the very core of helping them to wisely decide whether or not to start on a medicine. Obviously it is to our benefit to spend considerable time addressing the process that lies at the very center of this decision: "How do patients choose to take a medication?"

Curiously, one of the very best ways to most directly answer this question is to ask the question of the patients whom we, as physicians, know best – ourselves. Each of us has been a patient who, at one time or another, had to decide whether or not to start on a medication. In addition, most of us have been asked by friends or relatives what we think of certain medications, and many of us have had to decide whether one of our children should take a medication. Thus, we have a vast reservoir of direct personal knowledge about how humans of sound mind and reasonable intellect choose whether to take any given medication.

Our question is thus perhaps best reworded as, "How do we, personally, decide to take a medication?"

THE "CHOICE TRIAD"

In my workshops for primary care physicians, specialists, and mental health professionals, I have had the rare opportunity to ask the members of my audience the exact same question. The results have been remarkably similar. Physicians and nurses from all around the country tell me that they take medications for themselves if the following three criteria are met:

1. They feel that there is something wrong with them.
2. They feel motivated to try to get help with what is wrong (or to prevent future problems from arising) through the use of a medication.
3. They believe that the pros of taking the medication will, in the long run, outweigh the cons.

Nothing startling here. In all of the workshops I've given, I have never met a physician, nurse, clinical pharmacist, physician's assistant, or case manager who would ever take a medication (outside of "meds" such as vitamins or vaccines), unless they thought that there was something wrong and felt motivated to get help with the problem via the use of a medication. I have also never met a clinician who would ever take a medicine in which he or she thought the cons outweighed the pros. Why would any intelligent person do so? And so it is with our patients.

For ease of discussion we will refer to the three steps that a patient must navigate before trying a new medication (as well as staying on an old one), as the "Choice Triad." In the rest of the book, we will find ourselves repeatedly returning to this Choice

Triad, because an understanding of its nuances will provide a rich soil from which to transform our patients' hesitancies and fears about medications.

THE "GREAT DEBATE" IN ACTUAL PRACTICE

Now let us take a look at a very real patient in a very real setting, with a very real disease. How many patients in the middle of their first break of schizophrenia think that there is anything wrong with them? Having done this work for some 25 years, I can tell you – not many. So when a patient, perhaps a terrified adolescent boy of 19 years, tells me – "I am not going to take that medicine, Dr. Shea. No way. I don't need it. I don't want it. I'm not going to take it. And I can tell you where you can put it." – is he being resistant or oppositional in the sense of purposefully trying to antagonize me?

As we hinted at in our last chapter, I don't see why one would make that supposition; such a patient is seldom being oppositional. Instead, he believes, deep in his gut, without any hesitancy, that there is absolutely nothing personally wrong with him. He simply disagrees with me. Under these circumstances – a patient strongly disagrees with the first step in the Choice Triad – it would be quite foolish for the patient to take the medicine. It would not be a logical decision. Exactly like ourselves, if we did not feel that there was anything wrong, none of us would take a medication, especially an antipsychotic that could cause tardive dyskinesia and make our tongue dart in and out of our mouths like a lizard for the rest of our lives – so why should a patient do so?

I, personally, would never take a medication unless I felt there was something clearly wrong with me. In this instance, refusing the antipsychotic is not so much evidence of a person being illogical or oppositional as it is evidence of a person being prudent, if, indeed, he or she thinks that there is nothing wrong. The patient is making the exact same choice that I would make if I shared the same belief. It just so happens that in this case, I don't.

Once this insight is understood by prescribing clinicians, it follows suit that they develop a newfound respect for the patient's decision-making process – the same as their own – while not necessarily agreeing with the patient's database from which the decision was made or the decision itself for that matter. Our role becomes not one of making a so-called "resistant" or "oppositional" patient compliant but of helping a patient with poor information become better informed and motivated for change. We become teachers, and all good teachers are great motivators. Our goal is to increase our patients' genuine interest in trying a medication or staying on it after it has been started.

Over the years, I have found that once medical students, residents, and nurses truly understand the simple fact that patients refusing medications are often making the same decision that we would if we shared their belief set, it is rather remarkable how deeply it changes their attitudes toward "resistant" patients. More importantly, it changes how they come across to those patients who don't want to take medications. The oppositional feelings that trigger medication nonadherence described in the last chapter seem to melt away because the clinician realizes that the patient is making the wisest decision possible, given the belief set that the patient has at the time.

I am reminded of a quote by Armond Nicholi, Jr., a well-known psychiatrist who said, "Whether the patient is young or old, neatly groomed or disheveled, outgoing or withdrawn, articulate, highly integrated or totally disintegrated, of high or low socioeconomic status, the skilled clinician realizes that the patient, as a fellow human being, is considerably more like himself than he is different."[3]

Let us now take this reasoning much closer to home for the typical primary care physician functioning in a hectic clinic setting. Let us look not at a patient with schizophrenia – patients well known for refusing medications – but to a patient with diabetes.

We will look at a middle-aged woman, who is fairly symptom-free, except for unusually frequent daytime urination, nighttime

awakening with trips to the bathroom, and the recent onset of
a sensation of feeling weary. Moderately overweight and out of
condition, the level of her blood sugar suggests the need not only
of behavioral interventions such as diet and exercise, but also the
use of an oral hypoglycemic agent.

How many of these early diabetic patients starting on a long-
term medication ripe with potential side effects truly believe,
in their gut, that they have a serious disease on board, one that
can have crippling consequences and even have death as an end
point? Once again, I have had the luxury of asking many hundreds of primary care physicians this exact question during my
workshops. Even as I am phrasing the question, I frequently see
many physicians nodding their heads in agreement with the
point, because they quickly recognize that the answer is similar to the one that we observed in our patient suffering from
schizophrenia – that is, not many.

Indeed, patients whose diseases show minimal symptoms at first,
such as early diabetes or hyperlipidemia, are notorious for nonadherence. Early hypertension, where only an abnormal number magi-
cally culled from a blood pressure cuff is evidence of disease, may be
the king of nonadherence problems for just such a reason.

Sometimes, in my workshops, after the previous point has
been made by a member of the audience, a silence follows, and
then a physician will animatedly raise a hand, commenting, "I
have a caveat to that, though. The one set of patients with early
diabetes who fairly frequently do stay on their meds are those
patients who have a parent with severe diabetes or a friend
with it. You know, if their mom doesn't have a leg from the
knee down or their uncle has a pipe in his arm from dialysis,
those patients get it. They take the meds, and they often stay
on them almost religiously."

Thus, our point is made.

Exactly as our principles suggest, as outlined previously,
these patients will choose to start their medication because
they believe there is really something wrong with them. They
have a vivid picture of what could happen to them that moti-

vates them to try the medication, and they project that whatever the cons of this medication may be, it is probably not as bad as the potential dangers of their disease – renal dialysis, stroke, blindness.

The issue is not that these patients are smarter or less oppositional than our more typical patients with early diabetes, who refuse medications or who, more commonly, are poorly compliant with them. Simply, these patients truly believe there is something wrong. If they did not, they would not agree to taking the medication.

More importantly, if our "resistant" patients could be led to understand that there is something seriously wrong (i.e., they come to believe in the first step of the Choice Triad), there is a good chance that a large chunk of them will take us up on our recommendation for an oral hypoglycemic agent. They will have developed a sincere interest in the medication because of their personal belief (as opposed to our professional belief) that it could stave off serious problems. Patients take medications because of their beliefs, not ours.

FROM THEORY TO PRACTICE

Now that we have developed a better understanding and a sound theory, not only of the nature of medication nonadherence, but also of the internal thinking that leads to it, we need to put our theory to the test. As we stated earlier, a good theory will generate specific interviewing techniques and strategies that will help us to increase our patients' interest in both trying specific medications and staying on them. Will our theory do this?

To find out, let us return for a moment to the second step in the Choice Triad – the patient feels motivated to try to get help with what is wrong through the use of a medication. While discussing this second step in one of my workshops, a pediatrician who specialized in treating kids with asthma proffered the following tip, which I have found to be very useful.

INTERVIEWING TIP #1:   Inquiry into Lost Dreams

He commented that one of the most powerful motivators for these kids was the obvious one: They wanted symptom relief from their acute asthmatic attacks. But he had also found that there existed another very powerful motivator, that he could tap when his patients were having tough side effects or fears, that could help them to give their medications a little more time. He felt, and I have found with my own practice, that this same motivator was equally powerful for adults with many different diseases from rheumatoid arthritis to obsessive-compulsive disorder. What is this other powerful motivator that can help to transform nonadherence?

For many patients, it is not so much that they want relief from something the illness has given them (e.g., painful symptoms), they want back something the illness has taken from them – their dreams, their livelihoods, their peace of mind. The desire to recover what has been lost often provides an intense motivation to tolerate difficult side effects or to overcome the inconvenience or stigmata of taking medications.

The pediatrician described his interviewing tip as follows:

"I find it useful with my kids with asthma to ask them this question or a variation of it, 'Is there anything that your asthma is keeping you from doing that you really wish you could do again?' What I find with this age group is that there is often a quick answer to this question, and the answer is often related to a sport, say football or soccer.

"What I find to be so useful about this question is that it opens the door for adolescents, who by definition are prone to form oppositional relationships with adults, to tell me what they want me to do for them. They are calling the shots, not me. The oppositional field seems to dissolve away. Meanwhile, I gain a deeper insight into their motivation for seeking help from their asthma that goes beyond their desire for symptom relief. I might never have known this powerful motivator had I not asked. I can use this knowledge to enhance the adolescent patient's desire both to start a medication and to stay on it.

"First, although I never provide false hope, if I feel it is within reason, I can use this newly uncovered information immediately to help shape a shared agenda with a comment like, 'Now I can't promise this, but I have had some very good luck with helping other students, with asthma like yours, to get back into sports. We have some great meds that can help with that goal. Once again, no promises, but I would like to work with you to see if we might be able to get you back out on that soccer field. How does that sound to you?'

"Second, in the future, if there are tough side effects or if the stigma concerns so often seen with kids having to take meds at school become problematic, I can say something like, 'I know you are getting some tough side effects – and they are tough – but, fortunately, I have some ideas on how we might be able to make them much better, and I don't think we have yet seen the full power of these meds to help you feel better. We are still trying to get you back on that soccer field that we talked about in our first meeting. If you can give me another two weeks to see if I can lower the side effects and get you some better relief from these attacks, I think I might be able to do that. Is it a deal?'"

Very nice. Very nice indeed. Now *there* is a useful interviewing question – "Is there anything that your asthma (or whatever disorder is present) is keeping you from doing that you really wish you could do again?" – that can be used daily in the real world of a busy clinic to transform medication nonadherence.

The "inquiry into lost dreams" technique was developed directly from asking ourselves about ways of achieving the second step of the Choice Triad. Our model is beginning to show its power. Let us see what happens if we continue to explore the concept of improving motivation, which is, essentially, the heart of the second step of the Choice Triad. We have already seen that two powerful motivators exist: (1) relief from symptoms and (2) gaining back lost activities and dreams. Our next question is simple, yet potentially filled with great promise: "Are there other motivators we can tap for our patients?"

INTERVIEWING TIP #2:   Tapping Family Motivators

A primary care physician, during one of my workshops, shared a tip that I have found to be useful with many patients. His insight also touches upon the usefulness of understanding cross-cultural sensitivities when discussing medication interest. Much of his work was with the Latino population. He found that Latino men often do not want to take care of their disorders, because "taking care of oneself" is viewed as being self-centered. On the other hand, the Latino culture places a profound emphasis upon family ties and responsibilities, which displays itself as an intense belief in taking care of one's family no matter what the cost; family needs first, individual needs second.

Whether discussing diabetes, hypertension, or depression, he would try to become familiar with the patient's unique family history, family network, and sense of familial responsibilities. He would then tap this information to design an individualized strategy for motivating his patient.

For instance, let us say the patient lost his father, who had diabetes, to a myocardial infarction at age 51, and that the patient had found this experience to be devastating to him as a child. The physician might proceed as follows:

"Mr. Perez, I know you don't feel much like taking these medications for your diabetes, and I understand that. There might be another reason, in addition to taking care of yourself, why it may be very important for you to try to take them. I think they can help you to take care of your family. You see, your dad's diabetes is what led to his dying from a heart attack at such a young age. These medications can help to make sure that you don't get a heart attack, something that you know from your own experience would be horrible for your wife and kids. We need to keep you healthy, for them. I know it's a nuisance to have to take medications, I really do. I sure don't enjoy taking medications myself, but if it can save your family from that kind of pain, I think it is worth it. What do you think?"

A lovely tip. As an answer to our question, I believe that we have found a third powerful motivator for many patients – their families – that taps a deep-rooted sense of love and responsibility. This technique can also be expanded beyond family members. For some patients it is their commitment to their communities and to helping others that stands as a powerful motivator for them to stay healthy and capable of helping. As one would expect, this tip is also of great use, not only among the Latino population, but also across all cultures when we find individuals with a high sense of responsibility to family or mission.

Ed Hamaty, a pulmonologist from Philadelphia, added that such family or community motivators can be enhanced significantly by helping patients to create individualized affirmations such as, "This one is for my grandchild." A simple repeating of this affirmation every time the patient reaches for his or her medication bottle can go a long way toward inspiring motivation.

INTERVIEWING TIP #3: Providing a Visual Reminder for Family Motivation

A primary care nurse from Kansas, Janet Brack, suggested a wonderfully effective extension of this interviewing technique. Her tip moves us into the realm of nonverbal promoters of medication motivation. She noted that in smoking cessation programs it is not uncommon to ask participants to place a picture of a loved one on the cigarette pack itself to remind them of one of the reasons they are trying to kick the habit – to make sure they are still around to laugh, love, and help their families.

She asked herself, "Why not transfer this technique to the task of improving medication adherence?" She did, and she was impressed with the results:

"Mr. James, we've already decided that one of your reasons, besides taking care of yourself, that you want to stay on your medications for your high blood pressure is to keep healthy for your wife. That's a great goal, and I think you can do it. Some of my patients with a similar goal have found a neat trick to remind them why they are taking their medications. You simply set your pill bottle on a large picture of your family, so that every time you reach for it, you are reminded of what the losses may be to your family if you got a heart attack because of your high blood pressure. Many of my patients say it really helps them to stay motivated. How does that idea sound to you?"

THE MISSING PIECE OF THE PUZZLE

As we have moved from theory into practice, the power of our model is beginning to emerge. All three of the interviewing techniques that we have just developed – from our understanding of the second step of our Choice Triad – are simple, take little time, can be readily named, and can be easily taught to medical students, nurses, residents, and case managers. We are developing a model that provides concrete interviewing techniques and strategies that can be of practical use to clinicians as opposed to vague principles, such as "empower your patient," that offer little guidance as to the actual method of achieving in practice what is, in theory, undoubtedly an important goal.

One piece to the puzzle is missing: We need a word to talk about patient nonadherence, that follows our model and does not set up, by its very connotation, an oppositional feeling toward the patient, an oppositional feeling that the word *noncompliance* and, to a lesser degree, *nonadherence* seem to generate. In short, we need a name for our model.

REFERENCES

1. Cushing, H. Life of Sir William Osler. Oxford: Clarendon Press, 1925.
2. Holmes OW Sr. From address to the Massachusetts Medical Society, 1860.
3. Nicholi AM Jr. The therapist-patient relationship. *The Harvard Guide to Modern Psychiatry*. Cambridge, CA: Belknap Press of Harvard University Press; 1978:28.

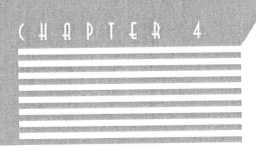

Is It Really "Noncompliance"?

"Words make a difference. The terms compliance and adherence should be abandoned because they subtly exaggerate the importance of the clinician, describe behavior inaccurately, and shed little light on motivations."[1]

John Steiner, MD, MPH

Mark Earnest, MD

Annals of Internal Medicine, June 2000

THE TROUBLE WITH THE WORDS *NONCOMPLIANCE* AND *NONADHERENCE*

As we begin to look for a word to describe our model, it is obvious that we need a word that allows us, in a nonpejorative way, to acknowledge that the number one cause of treatment failure is that many patients don't take their medications as prescribed, and they get sicker because of it. From the beginning, we have been emphasizing that one of the critical, perhaps the most critical, first steps in increasing medication use is the need to build a collaborative alliance with our patients, to create an atmosphere of "going with" them as allies against their illness, as opposed to "going against" them as antagonists to their beliefs. This nonoppositional stance is at the very heart of our philosophy and hence must be at the heart of what we choose to call our model.

In addition, it would be useful to find a term that emphasizes the collaborative spirit of the alliance, not just between the patient and the physician, but also among all of the parties involved in the battle against the patient's disease. Today, this treatment alliance may include a surprising number of diverse members, including the patient, his or her family members, the prescribing clinician (whether this be a physician, nurse clinician, physician assistant, or clinical pharmacist), the nurses, social workers, and pharmacists involved in ongoing care, and the case managers (who are becoming pivotal members of the treatment team in patients with diseases such as asthma, diabetes, congestive heart failure, bipolar disorder, and schizophrenia).

Unfortunately, as John Steiner and Mark Earnest note in our opening epigram, the most commonly used terms, *compliance/non-compliance* and *adherence/nonadherence,* don't seem to fit the bill. Not only do they tend to set the stage for an oppositional field of communication, but they also have other inherent problems, as Steiner and Earnest succinctly state. To better understand these problems, it may be of use for us to take a brief peek at the history of these words.

Historically, there appears to be a long tradition of labeling patients, as opposed to their behaviors, as problematic. As Steiner and Earnest point out in their classic article, "The Language of Medication Taking,"[2] in pre-1960 research studies on noncompliance, patients were described as "faithless"[3] to the treatment programs or as "untrustworthy" and "unreliable."[4] Near this time frame the word *noncompliance* came into vogue, and it has set an oppositional tone ever since. Although a good deal less castigating than *faithless,* the term *noncompliance* is hardly value-free.

One of the major problems with the term *noncompliance* is that it implies that physicians and nurses are the ones who make decisions on treatment and that patients are merely supposed to *comply* with these recommendations. Once again, we can see the power of language to set up, insidiously, the feeling of "going against" as opposed to "going with" our patients. But there is more to the problem, because these words also suggest that physicians have more control over medication use than they really do in actual clinical practice.

For example, the term *compliance* seems to suggest that physicians choose the medication, and then all that is left to do is to make sure that the patient complies with the physician's choice. But, as we saw in the previous chapter, physicians do not choose medications; patients do. Also, as the sociologist Peter Conrad[5] pointed out, not only do patients choose which medications they want to take, they also decide exactly how they are going to take them, a process Conrad aptly calls the patient's "medication practice." In the end, he points out that the only medication practices that count are those practices that patients choose to do, not the medication practices that physicians tell them to do.

The only time that a clinician indirectly controls medication practice is if the clinician literally hands the medication to the patient and watches the patient swallow it, as might occur on an inpatient unit. The only time the clinician directly controls both medication choice and practice is through the forced administration of medications via an involuntary commitment. Otherwise, concerning medication choice and dosing, the patient holds the cards. Before the patient walks out of our offices, it is to our advantage to see how he or she intends to play them. The term *compliance,* with its misleading suggestion of physician power, makes this simple truth too easily forgotten.

Another problem with the term *noncompliance* is that it is too generic, often yielding an inaccurate picture as to why the patient is not taking a medication. As we have seen, *noncompliance* has a not-so-subtle pejorative tone, yet it is often casually applied, not only to that small percentage of patients who may be purposefully oppositional – perhaps as the result of a personality disorder – but also to patients who forget easily, do not have enough money for the medication, are genuinely afraid of the medication, or simply do not think that there is anything seriously wrong with them or, if they do, do not feel that the pros outweigh the cons. Similarly, patients who miss a dose twice a week are grouped together as being "noncompliant" with patients who almost never take their medication.

According to sociologist James Trostle,[6] in his provocative article, "Medical Compliance as an Ideology," various alternative terms have been suggested to replace *noncompliance*, such as *nonadherence, defaulting, self-regulation,* and *self-management.* Others have suggested distinguishing those situations in which the patient has decided against medications because one of the beliefs in the Choice Triad has not been met (*intelligent noncompliance*) versus those patients who refuse medications solely for oppositional reasons (*capricious noncompliance*).

In my opinion, none of these terms seems to have "caught on" with busy front-line clinicians, whether in primary care or mental health settings. Perhaps the best of the lot, *nonadherence,* is generally the most commonly used in the parlance of today. At one level, *nonadherence* is certainly less oppositional sounding than *noncompliance* but still seems to lack appeal to many clinicians, perhaps because it sounds more like we are discussing the qualities of a roll of scotch tape than the intricacies of a therapeutic alliance. For many clinicians, *nonadherence* simply sounds sterile, cold, and uninviting.

Ideally, I think that we will want to find a term that highlights not the oppositional beliefs that can arise between the physician and the patient but the shared goals that they both embrace – finding symptom relief and, if possible, a cure for the disease. It should be a term that emphasizes that the goal of the clinician is not to choose the medication for the patient but to help the patient make a wise choice, which might even include the choice to not take the medication in the first place. Otherwise, we risk making our patients feel that they are being pressured to take *our* medications, not guided to choose *their* medications.

As one can imagine, I have spent more than a little time trying to find a word that effectively captures the above principles. I should admit up front that I have not always been totally successful in this quest. For instance, some years ago I had the brilliant idea to capture the model not with a single word but with a more comprehensive catchphrase, because there seemed to be so many important facets to the approach. The result read like this: *Non-Oppositional Nonadherence Strategies: Empathy, Nonjudgement, Sensitivity, and Engagement.*

At first glance, I was rather pleased with this catch phrase, because it seemed to summarize my key points while satisfying my more than ample compulsive psychological needs. However, when I shared it with my wife, who astutely edits all of my work, I could tell by her frown that she was not overimpressed. She commented, "I don't like it for three reasons: (1) It's too wordy, (2) It doesn't exactly roll off the tip of the tongue, and (3) Its acronym is the word NONSENSE.

Hmm. Good points.

Fortunately, a better term can be used to address the traditional problems housed under the name *noncompliance.* To find this term it is useful to look at our fourth interviewing tip.

This tip was provided by a primary care physician during a workshop in Minneapolis. She is describing one of the ways that she introduces her role as a physician to a patient during the part of their initial appointment when she is making her first medication recommendation. She reported that many patients seem particularly comfortable with this approach, and I certainly find it appealing. But in addition to being a nice model of one way of fostering a sound therapeutic alliance early on, it also holds the word that we are looking for as a descriptor to our model. We will present this tip exactly as if the physician were speaking to the patient.

INTERVIEWING TIP #4:   Introducing Medication Interest

"My goal as a physician is to always give you my best advice, whether that advice is to start a medication, stay on it, or get off it. Together we want to find a medicine that you are genuinely *interested* in taking because it makes you feel better. You're the one who is putting the medication in your body so it's your opinion that is most important, not mine. So please always let me know exactly what you think about the medications we are trying. I'm counting on your input. You know your body better than I do. And I think we can be a great team in finding a medication that works well for you – that really makes you feel better. How does that sound to you?"

With a single elegantly effective statement – "Together we want to find a medicine that you are genuinely *interested* in taking because it makes you feel better" – the physician fosters both a sense of collaboration and spotlights the goal that such a collaboration can achieve – relief from suffering.

The Missing Piece of the Puzzle Found

Equally important, we have stumbled upon the exact word that, over the years, I have found to be not only a nice descriptor of our model but also a practical replacement for words such as *compliance* and *adherence*. The principles that we have been describing, so far, in this book have come to be known as simply the *medication interest* philosophy and their application as the medication interest model.

In my workshops over the past seven years, physicians have given a warm reception to the term *medication interest*, perhaps because it emphasizes a point, well acknowledged by veteran clinicians, that one of the main skills of a successful physician is the ability to teach. Bottom line, we are teachers, we are motivators. Our successes depend directly upon our ability to find an effective medication (or an effective nonpharmacologic treatment) and then to motivate the patient to take it, by securing all three steps in the Choice Triad. Our treatment failures come from our failure to do so.

With a sense of shared exploration, we help our patients achieve an understanding that there is something wrong and identify what it is, motivate them to try a medication to help relieve what is wrong, and help them to weigh the complex pros and cons of the specific medication in question. After they have carefully weighed the pros and cons, the medication interest model views patients as capable partners, who, if their interest becomes high enough, will, ultimately, cross a threshold of interest that leads them to try the medication that we are suggesting, not because we tell them to, but because they believe in it – and in us. The term *medication interest* emphasizes that the real goal of prescribing clinicians, no matter what their discipline, is to increase understanding and motivation.

Our case management team found that we could completely eliminate the terms *noncompliance* and *nonadherence,* exactly as Steiner and Earnest suggested in our opening quotation, by simply referring to the patient's level of medication interest.

Instead of using oppositional terms, such as noncompliance and nonadherence, we would ask each other questions, such as the following:

1. How interested is Jim in taking his medication? (followed up with a question that provides a concrete idea of the level of interest, such as, "What percentage of the doses do you think he is actually taking?")
2. If he were here, how would he list the pros and cons that have led to his low interest?
3. Is his low interest related to the first, second, or third step of the Choice Triad?
4. Does anybody have any ideas how we could increase his interest?
5. How interested is his family in his taking the med?

In addition to asking questions, we also found that during our treatment team meetings, the word *interest* was effective in helping us phrase our answers to those questions in a nonjudgmental fashion with statements such as, "I think he is reasonably interested, but he is genuinely having trouble remembering the nighttime dose," "At one level he is clearly interested, but the bottom line is that he is simply frightened of the orthostatic dizziness. He is really worried that he'll fall and break his hip, which, at one level, is a reasonable worry," and "I think the problem with the interest here is a lack of money, and it's a genuine problem."

Moreover, in sharp contrast to my first shot at a catchphrase for our model (Non-Oppositional Nonadherence Strategies: Empathy, Nonjudgement, Sensitivity, and Engagement [NONSENSE]), *medication interest* seems to roll off the tongue rather nicely. It also allows us to discuss openly and frankly the main roadblock (i.e., not taking medications) to our patients' healing in a fashion that has no pejorative quality or oppositional bias to it.

We have found our final piece to the puzzle – a reasonable title for our model (i.e., "medication interest") – which is both a philosophy toward building the therapeutic alliance and a model for how to do so. We are now ready to put this philosophy and its model to the acid test. In our last chapter we saw how the model could help us develop specific interviewing techniques. Let us now push the model to see whether it can also develop complex interviewing strategies composed of multiple steps.

INTERVIEWING TIP #5:   Exploring Med Sensitivity

Few encounters are more critical in establishing alliances with our patients than our first meetings, and few moments are more treacherous to their development. The success of the first encounter can be more assured if we keep in mind that two opinions exist about every medication prescribed: the physician's and the patient's. With regard to whether the medication ever leaves the bottle, in the final analysis, only the latter opinion counts.

Even more importantly, patients not only have an opinion about the specific medication that we are prescribing, but also they have opinions about medications, in general, forged by their histories with previous prescribers and previous medications. As one can well imagine, sometimes these opinions are positive and sometimes they are not.

Thus, each patient arrives at our office for a first appointment with a certain degree of attitudinal "baggage" in tow. This baggage will often shape the patient's level of interest in our first prescription. Consequently, when we take our medication histories, it is not only useful to find out what medications have been ordered (and at what doses and for how long), but also what have been the patient's attitudes toward taking those medications.

In this light it can be argued that one of the most important questions to ask during a medication history is, "Do you take your medications as prescribed?" because the answer undoubtedly determines whether or not the medicines that we are about to suggest will be given a fair chance to help (or even be tried in the first place). The art is how to ask this question in such a manner that it is engaging, not challenging, in nature.

Let us see whether our medication interest model can provide some guidance on how to proceed. Keeping in mind that we want to minimize any phrasing that causes even subtle hints of opposition, the previous question may be too socially blunt, almost accusatory in tone, for many patients. It is probably ill-advised. To figure out how to phrase the question in a less oppositional manner, it may be useful to examine the patient's perspective on it.

Here is where it gets intriguing, because our question, "Do you take your medications as prescribed?" is often mirrored by a quite different question on the patient's side of the stethoscope: "Is this guy going to overmedicate me?" The latter question frequently arises from an ingrained opinion that previous physicians and prescribers have "overmedicated me, because they just don't get how sensitive I am to medications." It is an opinion that, for many patients, is deeply held. In fact, it is often an entrenched conviction garnered from decades of "bad experiences" with prescribing clinicians.

From the perspective of the medication interest model, it is a smart question for patients to ask, because it allows them to address the third step of the Choice Triad directly. If the medication is given at too high a dose for their bodies, bad side effects will indeed occur. The cons will outweigh the pros. From an intelligent consumer's perspective, it would make good sense to consider not filling such a prescription or, if filled, to take the medicine at a lower dose than recommended.

In short, if patients feel that the answer to their question is "yes," – we are going to overmedicate them – they are primed to have little interest in our medication recommendations from the get-go. The problem is that very few of our patients directly ask this critical question, because, like our own question, it is socially awkward. Consequently, they are forced to intuit whether we might overmedicate them, which is not a good state of affairs, because their intuition, perhaps primed by bad experiences with previous prescribers, may be very wrong indeed. An effective and reliable way exists to get around this potentially fatal trap to engagement.

Our model suggests that, paradoxically, the key to uncovering valid answers to our question, "Do you take meds as prescribed?" may well be to first answer the patient's question, "Do you overmedicate?" Only after the patient feels safe about this issue are we likely to get valid answers to our question or, for that matter, to trigger interest from the patient in our medication recommendations. Specifically, we want to demonstrate that we possess a keen interest in their concerns about side effects and, even more particularly, their views as to their medication sensitivity. The question becomes, "How?"

The answer may lie in a simple, but surprisingly useful, question that I ask after taking my standard medication history during an initial interview. Note that I often personalize it by using the patient's name. See what you think: "Mrs. Jenkins, do you think that you are particularly sensitive to medications?"

The answers are occasionally fascinating and, almost always, useful. If the patient quickly answers, "No, not particularly," then we have a "green light" to proceed with our initial medication recommendations. But, if the patient answers "yes" or indicates nonverbally through broken eye contact, tone of voice, or a pause before answering, then we have a "red light."

The light will not turn green until we sensitively uncover the patient's concerns and address those concerns to his or her satisfaction, a process that, in itself, will convincingly demonstrate that we have no intention of overmedicating him or her. Paradoxically, we will have answered the patient's question by asking one.

If the patient says that he or she is very sensitive to medications (and a good number of my patients emphasize, "I'm *very* sensitive to medications"), then it is common sense to follow up with an exploration of that patient's potential sensitivity with a question, such as:

> "What are some of the things that you have seen in the past with medications that has shown you that you are oversensitive?"

Such a question not only conveys our genuine concern, but also it can dig up all sorts of interesting information. In some instances, we discover that the patient does indeed seem to experience an overabundance of side effects, perhaps suggesting that the patient is a slow metabolizer. This information is invaluable in setting an appropriate initial dose so as to minimize side effects while maximizing medication interest and safety.

On the other hand, as I am sure you have seen in your own practices, we sometimes discover that a number of patients who view themselves as particularly sensitive to medications are, in truth, not. They simply encounter the typical side effects seen with medications of the class in question and, mistakenly, view themselves as being more side-effect prone than other people.

Obviously, with such patients, their inaccurate view of being "unusually sensitive" to medications will cast a considerable damper on their medication interest. In the past, I saw this as an opportunity to provide some productive education to counter this misinformation. I might say something like, "Mrs. Jenkins, I have some good news for you. In actuality, you aren't really overly sensitive to medications. You are simply getting very common side effects we see with those types of meds. Thus, we can try some other meds, and you may not get many side effects."

My hope was that by clearing up Mrs. Jenkins's misperception of being biologically overly sensitive, I would increase her interest in trying subsequent medications. Sometimes this happened, but many times, it did not. To my puzzlement, the "Mr. or Mrs. Jenkinses of the world" did not seem overly impressed by my well-intentioned educational foray, and, if their frowns were any indication, they were not particularly pleased with it.

Here is where the medication interest model suggests not only what to say, but also what might be best not to say. Keep in mind that we are discussing our first encounter with a patient. According to the medication interest model, the single most important thing to achieve by the end of the interview is that the patient feels allied with us. Any feelings of lingering opposition as the patient walks out the door, may be fatal to the filling of our first prescription and may undercut the likelihood of a return visit as well.

With these ideas in mind, let us look at what – beneath all my well-intentioned verbiage and intentions – Mrs. Jenkins may be actually "hearing" as I provide the educational information described above.

Physician: Mrs. Jenkins, do you think that you are particularly sensitive to medications?
Patient: Yes, definitely.
Physician: Well, I don't (*patient's eyes get big*). In fact, I have all sorts of other medications I'd like to try (*eyes getting even bigger*).
Patient: Okay (*patient thinking, God help me! He's going to overmedicate me like all the others*).

If we are honest, this is exactly what some of our patients are actually thinking at the time, and "it don't bode well" for medication interest. From the perspective of Mrs. Jenkins, I have asked for her opinion. She gave it. I ignored it. Then I told her that I had intended to ignore it.

"Hmm. I think I might be in a bit of trouble here."

Our model clearly suggests that this may not be the most effective direction to be taking in the initial meeting. But what direction might be better, keeping in mind that Mrs. Jenkins may be convinced by years of bad experiences with meds that she is overly sensitive?

For a moment, imagine that I simply acknowledge her opinion that she is overly sensitive to medications (noting to myself that in future sessions, once we have developed a stronger alliance, I might be in a better position to transform it). Further imagine, that near the end of the first appointment (if it is medically appropriate and safe), after I have written the name of the medication on my first script, I pause, look up at the patient and say something like:

> "Mrs. Jenkins, would it be okay with you if I start you off at one half of the recommended starting dose for this medication because of your concerns about being sensitive to meds? I think this would be a smart way to start you off. I call this a *baby dose* of the med, and I think it is a very gentle way to begin medications. This way, your body can get a feel for the med first before we give you much of a dose. Any side effects, and there might not be any with this little dose, will probably be much smaller in nature. Then when you are feeling comfortable on the medication, we can slowly increase it to get you feeling better and better. I just think this is a smart way for us to start. What do you think?"

Looks good on paper and, in practice, I have been pleasantly surprised just how effective the interviewing strategy of "exploring med sensitivity" can be in both spotting patients who have concerns about medications and in allaying those concerns before the first encounter ends. A patient, such as Mrs. Jenkins, who enters my office having been wary of physicians for years, may now leave my office feeling that she is in safe hands.

One can easily picture upon her return home, Mr. Jenkins asking his wife, "What did you think of Dr. Shea?" and her replying with an unexpected, "You know, he's the first damn doctor who ever listened to me." Here we have a nice example of a set of behaviorally defined interviewing techniques that have been woven together into an effective strategy for enhancing alliance while increasing medication interest.

For the technique to work most effectively, several things are worth noting. It seems to be important to "ask permission" at the end of the strategy, as reflected by my words, "What do you think?" because such a question further re-enforces our desire to work as a collaborative team. Telling patients why we are recommending a low dose (as a response to their concerns about being overly sensitive) is also important, because it conveys that we are not only carefully listening to the patient's input but also demonstrates that we are willing to act upon it, a point not missed by the patient.

THE PROMISE OF THE MEDICATION INTEREST MODEL

Our model seems to be working. It not only can generate specific interviewing techniques but also more sophisticated interviewing strategies. These strategies can be operationalized, named, taught, learned, and easily used. For instance, "exploring med sensitivity" is a simple four-step strategy:

1. At the end of a standard "medication history" in an initial H&P the clinician asks, "Do you think that you are particularly sensitive to medications?"
2. If the patient answers "yes," the clinician asks, "What are some of the things that you have seen in the past with medications that have shown you that you are overly sensitive?"
3. If the patient has the misperception that he or she is overly sensitive, the clinician does not challenge it.
4. When writing the first prescription, the clinician asks the patient whether it is okay to start the medication at one half its recommended starting dose and tells the patient why the recommendation is being made.

We have spent considerable time discussing the strategy of exploring med sensitivity, because it represents a nice prototype for many of the tips that will appear in the following pages. Hopefully, it also provides a convincing demonstration of the power of the medication interest model to generate specific interviewing strategies that may be of immediate use in our everyday practice.

Equally important, it shows how we can use the medication interest model to uncover new interviewing techniques based directly upon our years of clinical experience. The new tips that we develop by tapping our own clinical experience may prove to be particularly resonant with our personal interviewing styles, especially useful with a type of patient common to our particular practices, and, undoubtedly, worthwhile to pass on to the younger clinicians that come our way.

I believe that our model also holds great promise in the training of medical, nursing, clinical pharmacy, and physician assistant students. Imagine if medical and graduate schools assembled several educational packets of five or so interviewing techniques and the faculty told students, "No one is saying that these are the *right* way to talk with patients about meds, but our faculty feel that these are *reasonable* ways and have found them to be effective in their own practices. Consequently, before you leave our program, we want you to understand how they work and be able to demonstrate that you know how to use them." After their subsequent training in the techniques, each medical or graduate student would be asked to demonstrate the techniques with real or role-played patients before a faculty member. The results could be remarkable.

Finally, and, perhaps most exciting, is the fact that this model generates interviewing techniques and strategies that can be "tagged" and operationally defined. The result is that techniques and strategies can be quantified and empirically studied. We could train specific clinicians in a set of these techniques and then compare the rate at which their patients took their medications before and after the training.

In this fashion we may be able to demonstrate empirically that some interviewing techniques and strategies work more effectively than others. At that juncture we will have taken a large step toward developing an evidence-based model on how to talk with patients in ways that are more likely to enhance medication interest. Clinical science will have met clinical art with our patients being the benefactors. We will have proven what Steiner and Earnest said at the beginning of our chapter – our words do, indeed, make a difference.

REFERENCES

1. Steiner JF, Earnest MA. Lingua medica: the language of medication-taking. *Ann Intern Med* 2000;132(11):928.
2. Steiner JF, Earnest MA. Lingua medica: the language of medication-taking. *Ann Intern Med* 2000;132(11):926–930.
3. Jenkins BW. Are patients true to t.i.d. and q.i.d. doses? *Gen Pract* 1954;9:66–69.
4. Dixon WM, Stradling P, Wootton ID. Outpatient P.A.S. therapy. *Lancet* 1957;2:871–872.
5. Conrad P. The meaning of medications: another look at compliance. *Soc Sci Med* 1985;20(1):29–37.
6. Trostle J. Medical compliance as an ideology. *Soc Sci Med* 1988;27(12):1299–1308.

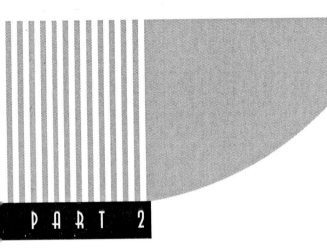

PART 2

Why Do Patients Choose to Stop Medications: **Three Key Questions**

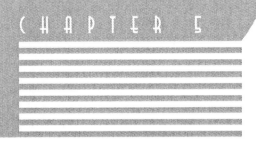

Outside the Office:
The Weighing of
the Pros and Cons

"Physicians are confronted by the particular souls of the
individuals and families before them. It is likely that much
noncompliance is an oppositional expression of an indi-
vidual's wish to be consulted and heard. . . . People want
to know that their opinions and concerns are worthy of
interest and response."[1]

Robert Shuman, EdD

from *The Psychology of Chronic Illness*

HOW THE PATIENT WEIGHS THE PROS AND CONS

We have seen how useful it has been to explore the nuances of
the Choice Triad, because it has provided us with a clearer understanding of how patients decide to try a medication. Each patient
must navigate all three steps of the Choice Triad – recognizing that
there is something wrong, being motivated to try a medication to
fix it, and deciding that the pros outweigh the cons – before a medication has a realistic chance of being taken on a regular basis.

By digging one step deeper into the patient's perspective, we
may uncover a treasure trove of new interviewing techniques. In

particular, if we turn our attention to the third step of the Choice Triad – the weighing of the pros and cons – we will discover remarkable differences in how individual patients go about this process.

Understanding this uniqueness is at the very heart of understanding how to increase medication interest, because there is a bottom line to medication interest. Even when a patient feels that there is something wrong and is motivated to do something about it via a medication, if that patient is not convinced that the pros outweigh the cons, the medication bottle will remain on the shelf. Period.

When we say that our patients are weighing the pros and cons, what exactly are they weighing? At the most basic sense, they are weighing beliefs. Each patient has a myriad of beliefs, some conscious, some unconscious, and many in between, about the medications that we are asking them to place inside their bodies. Robert Horne and John Weinman have done some wonderful work that helps to cluster these numerous belief sets. At its simplest level, they have found that patients "weigh their beliefs about the necessity of the prescribed medication for maintaining health now and in the future" with their "concerns about the potential adverse effects of taking it."[2]

Over the years I have found that most patients use three specific belief sets when placing their feelings and thoughts into the categories described by Horne and Weinman. Understanding these three belief sets can help us determine a more valid read on any given patient's medication interest, allowing us to address and often transform patient concerns before they become unfilled prescriptions.

The three different belief sets that determine whether a patient will stay on a medication once it is tried (or start it to begin with) are as follows:

1. Efficacy of the medication
2. Cost of the medication
3. Psychological meaning of the medication

Each of these three belief sets forms its own continuum. Each of our patients, as they are sitting on our examination tables or in our therapy chairs, has a position along these three continuums – toward one end or the other. For instance, concerning the efficacy of the medication, each patient has a personal belief about the extent to which a particular medication is "working." Some patients are convinced that the medication is helping a lot, whereas others are convinced that it is not helping at all. Of course, many are in between. But the closer the patient is to believing that the medication is not helping, the less his or her interest will be in staying on it. The point at which these three axes intersect gives us a good idea about whether the patient is about to stop the medication. Through these three belief sets, our patients decide whether the *necessity* of the medication outweighs their *concerns* about the medication.

Where the Patient Weighs the Pros and Cons

At this point our story starts to become a good deal more interesting and a great deal more practical, because much of what we have said so far is essentially common sense. But there is a catch to it.

A metaphor will help us understand the catch.

It is important to realize that few, if any, patients are sitting around, pencil in hand, making lists of the pros and cons. Patient beliefs are often a somewhat chaotic potpourri of opinions on numerous aspects of the medication from side effects to convenience, from cost to what the patient's partner and family think about the medication. These beliefs, some conscious, others preconscious, are all simmering in a stew from which a decision will emerge.

In a metaphorical sense, it is as if our patients have a committee inside their heads. Each member of the committee represents a differing opinion the patient holds about the medication. For instance, if the medication in question were an antidepressant, part of the patient might be saying, "This medication makes me feel better because it helps me stop crying." But another part of the patient might chime in, "Yeah, but I can't sleep on it." A third member of the committee might add, "But I can get back to work again." This positive vote may be quickly countered by another committee member arguing, "But this medicine is costing us an arm and a leg!" – And so on and so on, until it is as if the committee chair suddenly says, "We've heard enough, let's vote," And they do. The patient makes a decision – continue the medication or stop it.

Here is where the catch comes in: I have found that 90% of the time, when this committee votes – e.g. the patient decides to stop the med or continue it – the committee votes outside of my office. In short, the patient has either stopped the medication or has already decided that he or she does not like it before we meet again.

The problem is that if the committee votes outside my office, I do not get an opportunity to sway the committee before they vote. It's a done deal. And I generally find that if a patient has already stopped a medication, it is very hard for me to persuade the patient to try it again.

We are, by definition, important resources of information about medications for the committee, and, at times, strong lobbyists for their use. Patients value our opinions. Indeed, the more powerful our alliance, the more our opinions are valued. Perhaps the patient had some negative opinions about the medication that we could have helped with, as with a method of decreasing an unwanted side effect. Or perhaps the patient simply had some misinformation about the medication that we could have clarified very easily. In any case, we can do neither of these interventions if the committee has already voted.

A strategy now begins to emerge. It is a simple one. It is also one of the most important principles that I have ever found for maintaining medication interest – get the committee to vote inside my office. In short, I want to hear the patient's differing views on the medication while the patient is sitting in my office and, if possible, I want the patient to decide to stop or to continue the medication with me present. This effort has become one of my major goals during my med checks over the years.

The simplest way to accomplish this task is to directly ask for these opinions. Let us look at a prototypic example of the power of such direct questioning to uncover committee member beliefs, with a technique that I've found to be invaluable over the years.

INTERVIEWING TIP #6:   The Trap Door Question: Ascertaining
                        the Patient's View of the Current Dosage

As Robert Shuman so elegantly suggested in our opening epigram, patients want their opinions to be heard. Undoubtedly, one of the most important opinions that patients want heard, loud and clear, is their view on whether the dosage is too high. But all sorts of things can get in the way of this opinion being voiced or heard. The barriers are from both sides of the stethoscope.

From the patients' end of the stethoscope, they may have the misperception that we will be upset with them if they don't like the dosage that we are suggesting. In other cases, patients may lack the communication skills or assertiveness to spontaneously describe their hesitancies about the dose of the medication.

From the physician's end of the stethoscope, the problems are no less significant. One problem in particular is daunting – time – not enough of it. In the rush of the clinic flow, it is easy not to have time to sort out the patient's opinions, even one as important to hear as this one, if the patient does not spontaneously raise it. Also, unconsciously, we might not always want to hear it anyway, because if a patient does not want to advance a dose and is still sick, new interventions will need to be found and discussed. All of this takes time. It is so much simpler when the patient is thrilled with the medication and its dosage!

Along these lines, one of the most likely periods for medication interest to plummet to the point of discontinuation is when the physician – focusing upon inadequate relief of target symptoms – suggests increasing a medication to a patient who already feels that he or she is on too much but has not voiced that concern to the physician. If the physician then suggests the increase and the patient does not feel comfortable objecting, a large portion of such patients will likely have lowered or stopped the medication by the next session.

This phenomenon – patients not informing physicians that they are displeased with a dosage increase and then stopping the medication in the weeks after such an increase has been made – is so common that we have given it a name, the "trap door effect." The name comes from the fact that when this situation arises, the medication interest of the patient seems to disappear as if a trap door had opened beneath it, resulting in medication discontinuation.

The medication interest model suggests that it is wise to hear directly our patient's opinion on the current dosage – as opposed to assuming we know it – before making a recommendation to increase it. Thus, while performing a routine med check, in addition to wanting to know symptom severity, amount of relief, and side effects, we also want to uncover this critical bit of information. If, in a hectic clinic setting, I find myself about to recommend a medication increase when I don't know the patient's opinion on the current dose, I stop myself and ask the following particularly useful question:

"At this point in time, in your own opinion, do you feel that you are on too little, too much, or just the right amount of this medication?"

One of the strong points of this question is that it inquires along a continuum and thus does not bias the patient in any specific direction. You may discover, or may have already found, a question that works for you, perhaps with a slightly different slant. The important point is to directly ask for the patient's opinion about the current dosage before suggesting an increase. Assume nothing.

If the patient responds to the "trap door" question by sharing hesitancies or fears about the current dose, we now have an opportunity to address these concerns before proceeding with any suggestions for an increase in dosage. At times, the trap door question also uncovers a particularly problematic side effect, which, secondary to stigmatization, the patient had never shared, such as sexual dysfunction. In such cases, I can take actions to alleviate the side effect or may find it expedient to switch medications. I often find that patients know they are on the wrong medication before I do, and the trap door question sometimes helps me find out.

INTERVIEWING TIP #7:   Family Inquiry on Dosage

As we all know, some of the most influential lobbyists for or against the patient's use of a medication are the patient's family members. Spouses/partners may be particularly vocal. If you know that the patient's significant other is powerfully involved in the patient's care, a follow-up question along these lines may be of value:

"How does your spouse (or partner) feel about this dosage?"

If we are lucky enough to have the patient's significant other in the room, we can even more effectively collaborate, because the significant other may have legitimate concerns about side effects that the patient may tend to minimize. All sorts of side effects may have direct negative impacts on the patient's spouse/partner, including irritability, poor concentration, decreased sexual interest or performance, tremors, drowsiness, and weight gain. Because partners may see patients struggling on a day-to-day basis with tough side effects, they may also be indirectly affected by dosage increases: They become progressively more worried about their loved ones as the side-effect burden increases.

We are in the room to help the family as well as the patient, and it can be surprising – and refreshing – to a patient's significant other to turn to him or her and ask, "What do you think about this dose?" or "Are there any side effects that you have noticed that we haven't talked about that concern you?"

In this chapter we have looked at how a patient's "committee" decides to stop a medication and where, that is, *outside* our offices. In addressing these issues, we have uncovered the three belief sets that guide these decisions. In addition, we have looked at two tips based upon the medication interest model – one for the patient and one for the family – that demonstrate the power of direct questioning to uncover the views of the patient's internal committee members and external lobbyists before a vote is taken.

In the next three chapters we will find that it is well worth our time to explore individually each of the three belief sets that patients balance as they weigh the pros and cons. How patients arrive at their opinions within each belief set is surprisingly complex. Uncovering this complexity can help us avoid many other trap doors to medication interest, while uncovering even more ways to enhance the alliance with the patients who seek our help and the family members who are grateful for it.

REFERENCES

1. Shuman R. *The Psychology of Chronic Illness: The Healing Work of Patients, Therapists, and Families.* New York: Basic Books; 1996:92.
2. Horne R, Weinman J. Patient's beliefs about prescribed medicines and their role in adherence to treatment in chronic physical illness. *J Psychosom Res* 1999;47(6):555–567.

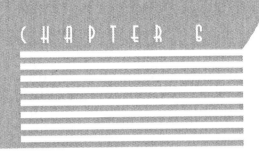

CHAPTER 6

A Question of Efficacy

"The most common rationales for altering medication practice are drug related: the medication is perceived as ineffective or the so-called side effects become too troublesome."[1]

Peter Conrad, PhD

FROM THE PATIENT'S PERSPECTIVE

As we continue to explore what makes patients interested in taking medications, we inevitably must examine the issue of efficacy, because efficacy is at the very heart of how patients weigh the pros and cons. Despite this fact, in over 20 years of clinical experience, I have yet to meet a patient who plopped into a chair in my office and commented, "I'm having some concerns about the efficacy of my Haldol."

For physicians the word *efficacy* has various technical connotations. From the patient's perspective, it is a good deal simpler. The issue of efficacy is often translated into the following straightforward question: "Does this drug make me feel better?" The patient's answer will frequently tip the scales one direction or the other with regard to medication interest.

As Peter Conrad suggested in our opening quote from his excellent article, *The Meaning of Medications: Another Look at*

Compliance, the answer to the patient's question, ultimately, comes down to whether the patient's perception of symptom relief outweighs his or her perception of side-effect damage.

From the view of understanding medication interest, the key word in the last sentence is *perception.* We often hear, both in research and clinical parlance, that a patient discontinued a medication because of a side effect. No patient has ever stopped a medication because of a side effect, unless the side effect killed him. Patients stop a medication because of their perception that the costs of the side effect are not worth the benefits of the medication, not because of the presence of the side effect itself. Side effects don't lead to discontinuation. Perceptions do.

By way of illustration, we all know patients experiencing severe side effects who stay on a medication nevertheless, because they believe that the effectiveness of the medication outweighs the cost of its side effects. To make our point in the primary care arena, we need only look at instances when patients tolerate the severe side effects of chemotherapeutic agents because they believe that the agents can save their lives. In psychiatry, patients with bipolar disorder in remission often tolerate the markedly unpleasant side effects of their antipsychotic agents and/or mood stabilizers, because these agents have rescued them from the ravages wrought by their manias and depressive episodes.

Returning to our metaphor from the last chapter, these patient perceptions represent positive votes in the patient's internal committee on medication interest. As we emphasized in that chapter, one of the main goals of any med-check, figuratively speaking, is to get the committee to vote in front of us. The art of securing this "in-house" vote lies in skillfully questioning our patients about their core beliefs regarding efficacy.

Interviewing Tips and Strategies for the First Appointment

We first encounter the power of this art when we navigate the interpersonal nuances of the initial H&P in primary care settings or the initial interview in mental health settings. During these opening gambits, we have an opportunity for establishing the trust with the patient that will enable the patient to openly share side effects in subsequent appointments. Without such openness, we may never hear the tell-tale signs forewarning imminent medication discontinuance.

INTERVIEWING TIP #8:   Introducing Physician Interest in Hearing About the Pros and Cons

Let us assume that we are meeting a patient for the first time, who is currently on various medications for asthma. The patient has already indicated some displeasure with his current medication regimen, but, overall, it has been helpful.

As we learned in Chapter 4, one of the fears that many – not all – patients bring to their initial appointment is that their new physician will overmedicate them or not take their side effects seriously. Such perceptions, if not addressed, may bias the patient to withhold medication concerns for fear that the physician will not want to hear them.

Many ways exist to address these fears. Once again, the following example is not proffered as the right way, but as an example of one way that you might find effective. Please feel free to pick and choose which approaches appeal to you personally, because each physician must find his or her own style of introducing medications. Moreover, each physician must learn methods for flexibly adapting that style to the unique needs of each patient. No matter which style one chooses, I believe it is useful to take the time to address the often hidden initial fears of the patient. I frequently use an approach very similar to the following. See what you think.

"I have tremendous respect for medications and have found them to be extremely useful in helping my patients. I just want you to know that I also realize that medications can have tough side effects, and I take those side effects very seriously.

"Personally, I only take medications when I feel that I genuinely need them, and I feel that the benefits outweigh the costs.

I take the same approach with my patients. So I won't suggest a medication unless I really have a feeling it will help you. I would never recommend a medication that I myself would not take or give to a member of my own family.

"And I always try to fill in my patients on possible side effects and the pros and cons of using the medication. You are currently on some excellent medicines, and there are some other excellent medicines out there. Our goal is to find the right combination that works best for you. How's that sound?"

Sounds good to me. I believe that introductions such as this one make it more likely that I am going to hear the voting preferences of the patient's committee members before the next vote is taken, before the medicine has been unilaterally stopped without my input. Thus, this interviewing tip provides another method of ensuring that the committee is more likely to vote inside my office not outside of it.

Asking for the patient's opinion at the end – "How's that sound to you?" – provides a nice touch that can provide insight as to how the patient has responded to this offer of a collaborative approach. Occasionally, a patient may be uncomfortable with such an approach, in which case, a modified approach with which the patient feels more comfortable can be developed.

For instance, some patients may become easily overwhelmed or frightened by too many facts and too many choices. These patients may prefer that the clinician provide a little less detail and a little more direction. The trick is to match the style of interaction to the needs and preferences of the patient, as opposed to the predilections and habits of the clinician.

In future appointments it will be equally important to find out in an ongoing fashion the patient's current perspective on the effectiveness of his or her medications versus the side effects. Paradoxically, the best time to set this stage is in the first appointment. In this regard, I might add a little later in our conversation something like this:

"By the way, if we run into any problems with side effects that lead us to think that the medication is causing more harm than good, I'll be the first one to tell you to get off of it. I'm not here to make you stay on any medication that isn't making you feel better or helping to control your illness in the long run.

"Our goal is to help you find a set of medications that you are genuinely interested in taking because they make you feel better, not because I tell you to take them. I'm always interested in your input, and I have a feeling we might be able to further help your asthma. . . . But fill me in for a moment. What has been your impression, overall, on how well your current medications are working out for you?"

This approach reassures the patient that we are here not only to tell them when a medication appears to be good for them but also to alert them when a medication appears to be bad for them. In some instances, the patient will be the first to be suspicious of such situations. On other occasions, we may be able to spot such a detrimental situation before the patient can because of our medical knowledge and experience.

No matter what the situation, patients feel much safer if they feel that we are friendly watchdogs keenly alerting them when to get off problematic medications. They feel much less safe if they feel that they need to be watchdogs keeping a wary eye on us, because they perceive that we may push them to stay on problematic medications. In addition, statements such as the previous one gracefully open the way for patients to share their views on their current medications.

Another point to remember during the introduction of a new medication, whether during a first appointment or with a well-known patient, is the value of expressing confidence in the medication.

INTERVIEWING TIP #9: Instilling Positive Expectations

We are not going to have the same confidence in all of our medications, and we should never feign confidence when we do not have it. But if you feel a medication has a good chance of helping, it is often useful to share that optimism with the patient. Keep in mind that all medications carry within them a potential placebo effect. This placebo effect is not something to be ignored; it is something to be enhanced. Placebo effects sometimes cure. In other instances, they may enhance the pharmacological efficacy of medications or independently change brain physiology by themselves, as has been seen in several antidepressant studies.[2,3]

If the prospective medication has demonstrated good results in well-controlled clinical trials, I go out of my way to let the patient know of this fact. I also find it useful to be specific about instances in which the medication has personally been valuable with my own patients. Such personal endorsements by me are often much more persuasive to patients than a horde of research studies. Fortunately, we can take advantage of both approaches as follows. Imagine for a minute that we are talking with a patient about one of the newer medications for congestive heart failure:

> "This medication has really proven itself in recent research, and I, personally, have had some great luck with it. I would say that in the last two months alone, I've had at least a dozen patients, sitting in that exact chair, who have had very significant improvements in their breathing and ability to get around since we started them on it. There are no guarantees, but it can be really pretty striking how much better people feel when taking it."

INTERVIEWING TIP #10:　The Talisman Effect: Optimizing the Power of the Prescription to Symbolize Hope

Our written prescriptions are not only sterile communications to pharmacists about medications, but also, for some of our patients, they are tangible symbols of hope. Curiously, from the perspective of cultural anthropology, prescriptions share some striking similarities to talismans, even to the point of being partially written in a secret language (Latin) that is understood only by the healers of the culture but not by those people seeking the help of those healers. I'm not suggesting that prescriptions are talismans, but I am suggesting that symbolically, like talismans, they may be powerful enhancers of the placebo effect in their own right.

As such, it may be useful, from a psychological perspective, "to charge them" with the power of our own belief. A patient with intractable pain, debilitating depression, or AIDS is looking for hope, even if the hope is for just a small relief in suffering. This is a hope that talented physicians sometimes enhance, not only by their choice of medications, but by how they handle the pieces of paper that procure those medications.

If I have a good feeling that a particular medication is going to help a patient, I have found it useful to do the following. As I hand the prescription to the patient, while we are both holding it, I explain the directions. After I'm done, I look the patient directly in the eye and say the following: "Well, good luck with this. I've got a really good feeling it is going to help you."

It is a simple gesture. It takes no time. But it is the type of gesture from which hope is sometimes born.

INTERVIEWING TIPS AND STRATEGIES FOR FOLLOW-UP APPOINTMENTS

So far, we have spent a great deal of time emphasizing interviewing techniques for use in the initial H&P or in the initial interview for a mental health professional. In our follow-up appointments, it is both critically important and surprisingly easy to show our continued interest in hearing about our patients' views on the pros and cons of their medications.

INTERVIEWING TIP #11:   Ascertaining the Patient's Ongoing
Views on Efficacy

We can see that patients generally possess beliefs on two different continuums regarding the efficacy of a medication: (1) the effectiveness of the medication to provide relief from symptoms and (2) the tendency of the medication to produce side effects.

With regard to effectiveness, each patient sits on a continuum ranging from "this medication really makes me feel better" to, at the other end, "this medication does absolutely nothing for me." Naturally, the closer the patient is to this latter end of the continuum, the closer the patient is to stopping the medication. Simultaneously, every patient has an opinion on the severity of the side effects, ranging from "I'm not getting any of those side effects Dr. Shea mentioned" to, at the other end, "I don't know what Dr. Shea was thinking, but I'll tell you one thing, he never tried this drug because it makes you feel like hell." Any patient near this end of the continuum is getting ready to discontinue his or her medication. In fact, if we were to plot these two continuums on the same graph, noting where they intersected, we would get a very good idea of how close the patient is to discontinuation.

This information is incredibly important, because it can allow us to intervene and perhaps prevent unnecessary medication discontinuance. Fortunately, there is no reason not to know this information, that is, where the patient sits on these two continuums, because most patients are eager to tell us if they are asked, but we have to ask.

Questions, such as the following, are effective at uncovering the patient's views on whether the medication's effectiveness is outweighing its side effects. One doesn't need to ask all of these questions. We simply pick and choose which questions may be most productive with any given patient:

1. How's that medication working out for you that we started up last time?
2. Is the medication helping with any of your symptoms?
3. Are you getting any of the side effects that we mentioned last time?
4. Are you having any problems that you are wondering whether or not they may be a side effect?

5. What do you think about the medication, so far?
6. Do you like the medication, so far?
7. Do you feel that the relief you are getting outweighs the side effects you are having at this point in time?
8. At this point in time, do you feel that the pros are out-weighing the cons with this medication?

If the patient is having side effects, it becomes important from a medical standpoint to ascertain their severity. From a medication interest standpoint – in an effort to uncover whether the patient is about to stop the medication – it is equally im-portant to see how the patient perceives the severity of the side effect. This perception is always unique to the circumstances of the patient. A dry mouth may be of minimal concern to a mason, but it may be a reason to discontinue the medication to a public speaker.

INTERVIEWING TIP #12:   Techniques for Conveying Concern
About Side Effects

Any or all of the following questions, some open-ended and some more directive, can help patients share their knowledge about the personal impact of their side effects from a psychologi-cal standpoint. For the purposes of illustration, let us pretend that our patient is experiencing dizziness:

1. Tell me about a specific time you felt dizzy and walk me through what happened.
2. Just how bad does the dizziness get?
3. How often are you feeling it?
4. How many days this week did you get it?
5. Is it making it harder for you to do anything?
6. On a scale from 1 to 10, with 1 meaning "it hardly bothers me" and 10 meaning "I can't stand this side effect," where would you put your dizziness this past week?

7. I have some ideas about what to do to get rid of the dizziness, but if we can't, do you think the dizziness is bad enough that it outweighs the good things your medication is doing, like making it easier for you to breath and getting rid of some of that swelling in your legs? Sometimes it's a tough call, but only you can make it. The bottom line is do you think you feel better on or off the medication at this point?

Such questions cut to the core of the matter so that there is no miscommunication possible here between the patient and the physician. By understanding how problematic a side effect is, we can help the patient weigh the pros and cons more effectively. Moreover, the reporting of side effects, perceived as severe by the patient, may be the harbinger of imminent medication discontinuation.

INTERVIEWING TIP #13:   Probing for Impending Discontinuance

If, during follow-up visits, a patient spontaneously raises concerns about a side effect, I have found that it is important to explore this side effect thoroughly. A spontaneously raised side effect often suggests that it is causing enough problems that the patient may be considering stopping the medication. In my experience, if a side effect is spontaneously raised several times, this medication is probably heading for the back shelf of the medicine cabinet. If we have any questions about the intensity of a patient's misgivings, here is the time to ask and here is an effective way to do it.

"Mary, we've been trying to decrease this side effect, but I know it is still a problem. What kind of thoughts, even fleeting in nature, have you had about maybe stopping the medication?"

I have been pleasantly surprised how, after using this technique, patients sometimes describe serious misgivings about the medication in question. This disclosure opens the door for a productive discussion of what to do for the side effects and whether to continue the medication without there being any shame or guilt for the patient about having had such thoughts. Once again, we are doing everything we can that will decrease any oppositional feelings between our patients and ourselves.

This technique leads directly into a discussion of our last interviewing tip for this chapter, which also has to do with decreasing shame and guilt while enhancing a collaborative alliance.

INTERVIEWING TIP #14:   Proactively Recommending
                                      Discontinuance

As hinted earlier, patients sometimes worry that we will be upset if they suggest stopping a medication. They fear that it may look like they complain too much or don't want to help themselves. If they project this fear on to us – despite the fact that we, personally, take their side effects very seriously – they may choose to say nothing. In such situations, it is often only a matter of time before they stop the medication on their own.

One nice way of nipping this problematic process in the bud is to remind the patient that we, too, are aggressively on the lookout for side effects. As mentioned earlier, part of our goal is to be a watchdog that alerts our patient when it may be best to stop a medication because the side effects are outweighing the benefits.

I have found no better way to convince a patient of my vigilance regarding side effects than to be the first one to suggest stopping a medication. When patients repeatedly raise a problematic side effect, one that could easily lead them to stop the medication, a response such as the following can go a long way toward reassuring them that we, too, share their concerns:

"Jim, I just don't like the problem we are having with this side effect. If we can't get it under control, I really think we may need to stop this med, even though I know it's also helping too. I'm just worried that the pros of using it are being outweighed by the cons. What do you think?"

I, personally, have found this technique – being the first one to proactively suggest stopping a medication – to be a very powerful tool. I use it a lot when dealing with side effects from antidepressants.

In this chapter, we have carefully reviewed the various beliefs that patients may have about the efficacy of their medications. Patients carefully weigh these beliefs and decide whether the medication's benefits outweigh its costs. If they don't, medication interest plummets, and the medication bottle sits idly in the medicine cabinet, or the prescription goes unfilled.

Clearly, the patient's views on efficacy described in this chapter play a major role in medication discontinuance but not the only role. As we noted in the last chapter, two other belief sets play a significant, sometimes determining, role of whether a medication ever makes it out of its bottle. Now is the time to look at one of them – cost – in terms of both money and convenience.

REFERENCES

1. Conrad P. The meaning of medications: another look at compliance. *Soc Sci Med* 1985;20(1):29–37.
2. Leuchter AF, Cook IA, Witte EA, et al. Changes in brain function of depressed subjects during treatment with placebo. *Am J Psychiatry* January 2002;159:122–129.
3. Mayberg HS, Silva JA, Brannan SK, et al. The functional neuroanatomy of the placebo effect. *Am J Psychiatry* May 2002;159:728–737.

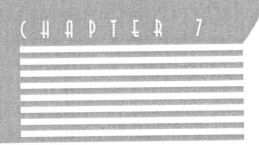

A Question of Cost

*"It may be argued that the ongoing personal relationship
with each patient is the . . . tool of the trade for the primary
care physician. The primary care physician's approach to
the patient's problem is grounded in the way the patient
defines the problem."*[1]

Howard Brody, MD

from *The Healer's Power*

First Things First: I Don't Have Enough Money to Get My Medications

Cost is the second major belief set that patients weigh while
deciding whether to continue or to stop a medication. Cost is
translated by most patients into a question such as "Is it worth it
to me to take this drug?" Somewhat surprisingly, if one lists by
frequency the reasons that patients do not take medications or
take them erratically, financial cost is not necessarily near the top.
On the other hand, when cost is the problem, it is often deadly
with regards to medication interest. Returning to our "internal
committee" metaphor, on the pro side the patient may have many
voices singing the praises of a medication, but all one needs is one
member of the committee to say, "That's all well and good, but
we simply don't have the money and that's that."

As clinicians, we need to know whether such a hostile vote is about to be cast by a committee member, and we need to know while the patient is in our offices, so that the medication is not axed two weeks from now, unbeknownst to us, because of cost issues. Such a discontinuation will, at a minimum, result in increased morbidity. At a maximum, it can result in increased mortality, as with a seriously depressed patient in which the antidepressant is keeping suicidal ideation at bay.

In some unfortunate situations, a hostile family member, as with an abusive spouse, may push the cost situation "over the edge" with comments, such as "I'm sick and tired of you and your depression. We all have to deal with stress. Do you see me reaching for a pill that costs a fortune? Do you have any idea how much strain your damn pills are putting on us financially? No, I wouldn't think you would. The only person important to you is you." For a patient on the receiving end of such a vicious diatribe, there will be a considerable psychological penalty paid for continuing on medication. It represents a legitimate con that could easily tip the scale toward stopping the medication.

We want to be aware of cost issues as a potential serious problem, not only because they can lead to medication discontinuance, but also because we may be able to do something constructive to prevent such discontinuance. Cost is a medication interest problem, though not always easily solved, that does have a surprising number of potentially helpful solutions, including use of generics, use of medication samples, formal use of pharmaceutical programs for indigent patients, and supplemental governmental programs.

More specifically, as Howard Brody stated in our opening epigram, we need to see how each patient is defining the problem of cost, because patients may be embarrassed by their financial situations. In such instances, instead of viewing money as the problem, patients view themselves as the problem for not having enough money. This type of negative self impression can make the topic of cost a taboo one. If we don't know of the problem, then there is nothing we can do about it. A nurse who happened upon my working on this manuscript in a café shared a tip that addresses this exact dilemma.

INTERVIEWING TIP #15: Gently Exploring Cost Issues

Her tip comes in the form of a simple admonition: Develop the habit of routinely asking every patient about the cost of his or her medications, because if you don't ask, you often will not be told. By demonstrating a matter of fact curiosity about the cost of the patient's medications, much of the taboo quality to the topic seems to fall away. As a physician, hearing about the costs of the medications that I am prescribing is also sometimes sobering, a realization that prompts me to more aggressively look for the most cost-efficient way to help my patient. Let us see this strategy at work:

"Mrs. Jackson, I'm always curious on how much my patient's medications cost. How much did you end up having to pay for the (insert medication in question) this past month?"

"Were you surprised by the cost?"

"How much of that did you have to pay for yourself?"

"It can be tough for anyone to pay for their medications; how much of a burden do you think this will be for you and your family?"

Routinely asking such questions assures insight into the cost issues potentially impacting on our patients' medication interest. Using these interviewing techniques the clinician can gently open the door into this critical topic.

Naturally, generic medications, of a certified bioequivalence, are a reasonable first answer. Another thing to keep in mind is that, especially with antidepressants, a pill that is twice the dosage of another one may be only fractionally more expensive. In such a case, if the pill is scored, you can write the script for pills of the double dosage and then instruct your patient to cut the pill in half, being sure that the patient is able to do so effectively. I sometimes have patients demonstrate in front of me how they halve the dosage to make sure that they can do it appropriately, keeping in mind that patients with rheumatoid arthritis or failing eyesight may have trouble with such a task.

On a more systems-wide perspective, with the hectic pace of our clinics, anything that slows up a physician, nurse clinician, or physician assistant is going to have a tendency to not get done. Sometimes a lot of chart culling and paper processing is needed to get a patient enrolled in one of the pharmaceutical plans for the indigent. If there are particular medications that you often use in your clinic that are available on such plans, it may be useful to have your office manager type up a list of those medications, including whom to call, the telephone number, and what information will be needed from the chart for that particular pharmaceutical company plan. Such a list posted on the wall of the examining office serves both as a prompt to consider such programs and as a much appreciated way of getting the job done quickly, with the least amount of hassle. The bottom line of such a posting is that more people may get the advantage of some of these remarkably generous pharmaceutical programs.

THE HIDDEN COST: INCONVENIENCE

The patient's answer to the question, "Is it worth it to me to take this drug?" is not always related to cost, in the sense of money. In the outstanding book, *The Doctor-Patient Relationship in Pharmacotherapy*, one of the contributors, James Ellison makes the following point that is often not given enough attention: "In general, patients should be discouraged from beginning a treatment that is likely to become burdensome as a result of inconvenience."[2] At first glance the point seems painfully obvious, but I have been surprised at how often I seem to ignore it.

I ignore it, not because I do not believe it, but because I am un-aware just how inconvenient this particular regimen for this particular patient has become, because I have not asked about it directly. As with financial cost, subtle taboos push patients toward silence on this topic. In this section we will explore some of those taboos and describe specific ways to remove them in actual practice.

Let us review the importance of inconvenience as a cost to the patient. No definitive data exist on this point, but I suspect that the cost to the patient, because of inconvenience, may well be a more frequent cause of decreased medication interest, or even medication discontinuance, than money. Inconvenience can manifest in may ways, and it often presents as a daily problem.

On a mild side, with a patient who is easily forgetful, multiple dosing schedules frequently result in missed doses. All of the hassles inherent in trying to remember when to take one's medication present as an ongoing and unpleasant inconvenience. On a more moderate side, a disabled or elderly patient may find it difficult to drive to the pharmacy. Sometimes the waits at the pharmacy are surprisingly punishing for a patient with congestive heart failure, who is uncomfortably short of breath, or a patient, with a social anxiety disorder, who is acutely intimidated by a crowded pharmacy waiting room. On a more severe side, a patient who must hide medication use from a boss who frowns upon "sick employees" may need to fret several times a day as he or she sneaks off to the bathroom to quickly gulp down a tablet or two. Even darker in nature is the patient with an alcoholic spouse who is highly opposed to medications and could erupt into physical violence if his wife's "dirty little secret" is revealed. With such severe concerns regarding the cost of inconvenience on board, the patient's internal committee may wisely answer the question, "Is it worth it to me to take this drug?" with a flat-out "no." As we have seen so many times before, the art is to help the patient share these concerns during the office visit itself.

Let us look at an example of one of these problems: an elderly woman who finds driving to the pharmacy to be frightening. She has a son who can do it for her, but he lives 30 minutes away. She feels guilty that he has to drive this distance to get the prescription from her and then drive another 15 minutes to the pharmacy. Our patient is between the proverbial rock and the hard place. She needs the medications. It is daunting to go herself. She does not want to inconvenience her son. If we remember the advice of Ellison, it looks like we are setting up a situation where inconvenience is going to become burdensome.

INTERVIEWING TIP #16:   Calling in Prescriptions for the Patient

While presenting a workshop at Riverview Physician Services in Wisconsin, a certified medical assistant provided me with a ready-made tip for this problem. She commented that with the elderly or disabled (or with anyone who had transportation problems), especially when writing the first script, she asks:

> "Would you like me to call that prescription in for you? Once I've called it in, you won't have to wait as long at the pharmacist and, if you like, someone else could pick up the medication for you. You can even call ahead and make sure the prescription is waiting for you."

She reported that these patients often seemed visibly relieved and were genuinely appreciative of this simple act of kindness. Not only had a potentially disengaging roadblock to medication interest been dismantled, but also the patient had found a clinician who cared.

THE SHAME CYCLE: A CURIOUS, YET PROBLEMATIC, COST OF INCONVENIENCE

People forget to take medications. It happens, even to the most motivated patients. How often it happens is related to both internal factors (how prone the patient is to forgetfulness, the presence of disorders, such as adult attention deficit disorder and dementia) and external factors (frequency of dosing, the pace of the patient's workday). Both internal and external factors combine to determine how inconvenient taking a medication becomes for any given patient.

But a third factor not often discussed – the psychological ramifications of missing doses – ultimately plays a significant role in how problematic the inconvenience becomes. These psychological ramifications shape the patient's perception of the severity of the inconvenience. If the patient experiences psychological pain for missing doses, inconvenience of dosing becomes a more significant issue, because with every missed dose the patient suffers.

The extent of this pain can be surprising. Sometimes it causes powerful damage to the patient's medication interest. It can also damage our therapeutic alliance to the point that a patient may drop out of care. This type of breakdown in therapeutic alliance is curious because of its paradoxical nature. Such a therapeutic rupture is most commonly encountered, and is most destructive, with clinicians who are particularly good at engaging patients. It also insidiously unfolds, essentially being invisible to the treating clinician and hence beyond intervention. Consequently, studying it in some detail is well worth our time.

The shame cycle occurs more frequently in patients who have low self-esteem, as seen with patients who have been abused, live with belittling partners, have poor life-skills and encounter a steady diet of failure, or are viewed as unattractive in their cultures. In short, the shame cycle is prone to occur in a lot of our patients.

Such patients often have an intense need to be liked and are exquisitely rejection-sensitive. Pleasing their doctors and to be perceived by them as "good patients" is unusually important to these patients. When such a patient finds a warm and engaging physician, they quickly bond. To the treating clinician, all seems to be going well; the physician likes the patient, and the patient likes the physician. The appointments are a pleasure for both parties, until . . .

Until one of these patients, perhaps a patient with more than a fair share of forgetfulness, begins to miss doses. These patients then experience shame and/or guilt, two emotions that are obviously unpleasant. But with patients who have been abused or are prone to self-denigration, shame and guilt are all-too-familiar points of intense pain. With these patients there is a psychological cost to missing doses. The frequency of this cost is directly related to the inconvenience of taking the medication. The shame cycle has begun.

Each time such a patient comes into our offices, the patient is fearfully anticipating a question from the clinician, along the lines of, "Mrs. Phillips, have you been taking the medication the way it is prescribed, you know, twice a day, once in the morning and once at night?" No matter how warmly this question is proffered, the patient is now faced with a dilemma – tell the truth and risk losing the respect of Dr. Shea or lie and risk losing self-respect. It is a lose/lose proposition. Sometimes the shame is so intense that the patient opts for the latter to save face. This path further stokes the shame cycle, because the patient now experiences a new shame related to the deception.

For these patients, there is now an insidiously unpleasant association occuring when "seeing Dr. Shea," despite the fact the patient views Dr. Shea as warm and caring. As more and more doses are missed, the shame cycle intensifies. In these situations, that the medication is being taken erratically is bad enough, but something much more serious is about to happen, that is, these patients are about to stop coming.

They stop because the intensity of the shame and guilt is too big a price to pay. For these patients, the cost of the inconvenience related to missing doses is too high, and it is no longer "worth it to them to take this drug." When the next appointment day comes up, it is all too easy to rationalize, "I've got a lot I need to do this week. I just have to get to the grocery store. I just don't have time to go today. I'll go to the next appointment." A missed appointment means more shame, more lying, more guilt, and more missed appointments. The shame cycle worsens. Soon enough our patient is a permanent "no show."

What is particularly frustrating is that the clinician has no idea that any problem is arising, and, consequently, can do nothing to transform it. I have found the following strategy to be useful in short-circuiting the shame cycle. See what you think.

INTERVIEWING TIP #17: Short-Circuiting the Shame Cycle

I implement this strategy in the first appointment, as I am introducing my approach to prescribing medications. It goes like this:

"It is very easy to forget to take a dose. If you notice yourself doing that, please note whether there is anything inconvenient about the timing of the dose. If there are any missed doses, we can put our heads together to see whether we can figure out a better time or an easier way to remember. The bottom line is that I really think this medication can help you, but I want to find a way that is easiest for you to remember to take it. Can you promise to let me know about any missed doses? And we'll see what we can come up with to make sure taking the medication is easier to remember. Is that something that you think you can do?"

What a nice antidote to the shame cycle. No shame here. Patients often model whom they think they are by whom they think we think they are. If when a patient misses doses, the clinician's tone is one that conveys displeasure, the patient will often adopt the image that he or she is at fault, that is, a bad patient.

In the previously described strategy, there is none of that. The physician views the inconvenience of the scheduling as the "bad guy" and the patient as the "good guy," whose input is vital. The patient is viewed not as the problem but as the solution. The strategy is a wonderful example of an effective application of the medication interest model. "Nonadherence" is seen not so much as something that the patient does but as an experience the patient and the physician share.

At the next session the physician asks, "Did you notice any problems with the doses being inconvenient or find yourself missing any of them?" With such words the discussion of missed doses opens up gracefully without a shred of shame or guilt. Sometimes patients have even kept a list of the missed doses. Such meticulous tracking can be positively re-enforced with, "You've done a great job of keeping track of the missed doses. It will really help us to find a convenient time for you to take the medication."

Suddenly, a patient who – without the use of our strategy for short-circuiting the shame cycle – would have been experiencing a negative experience for missing doses is – with the use of the strategy – having a positive experience for responsibly reporting the missed doses. The potentially oppositional field seen in the shame cycle has been completely reversed.

By the way, a lot of slick ways can help forgetful patients remember doses. Naturally, plastic pill cases, in which the day's doses are placed in separate compartments can really help, and they have the added advantage that one can readily see when a dose has been missed – the pills are still in the case!

Some of my favorite memory triggers rely upon making the presence of the medication bottles hard to miss by associating them with something that the patient never misses doing:

1. If the patient brushes his or her teeth daily, then I suggest placing the medication bottle right between the patient's toothbrush and toothpaste tube. It is hard to miss a dose with this technique, especially if you emphasize that the patient should take the medication before brushing his or her teeth.
2. Placing the medication bottle directly beside morning vitamins is also very effective. Care must be taken if children are in the house, that no confusion can occur, nor should potentially dangerous medications be out in such instances.
3. Yet another technique that some of my patients claim has worked nicely is to place the medication bottles on top of the pillow on the bed or on top of the alarm clock, two places that must be encountered every night before sleeping.
4. It is also useful to brainstorm with the patient's family on any novel ideas they may have on how to remind the

patient. Unique, creative, and, more importantly, very effective reminders sometimes come from such family brainstorming.

Of course there is one caveat to all of this excellent clinical practice. To help with missed doses, the clinician must know about them. We already saw, with short-circuiting the shame cycle, one approach that enhances the likelihood of uncovering missed doses. Here is another one; only this time, it is an interviewing technique designed for use during ongoing medication checks.

INTERVIEWING TIP #18:   Normalizing Missed Doses

Research by Steele and colleagues has shown that how physicians ask about missed doses plays a significant role in whether valid answers are forthcoming.[3] Their research also showed the troubling fact that only 12% of their patients spontaneously mentioned anything about how they were actually taking their medications. As we have seen so many times before, if one wants to know, one has to ask.

Here is a tip for eliciting more accurate information on missed doses that I have found to be very effective. It evolved from combining two interviewing techniques – "normalization" and "gentle assumption" that psychiatrists use to improve validity when uncovering sensitive or taboo material such as violence, incest, and substance abuse.[4] The cornerstone of the technique is twofold: (1) The process of missing the medications is normalized so as to decrease shame or guilt and (2) the clinician does not ask if medications were missed; it is gently assumed. When applied to the process of uncovering missed doses, it looks like this:

"Mr. Jeffers, many patients tell me that it can be easy to forget to take medications at times (normalization). In the weeks since we last met, how many doses do you think you might have missed per week, just roughly" (gentle assumption).

This interviewing technique works extremely well. You will have to see how it works for you, but I have a suspicion that you will be very pleased. I have seen clinicians inquire about missed doses with questions such as, "Have you missed any doses?" or "You've been taking the meds as we discussed?" and receive assurances that all medications are on board. A second clinician, during a later interview, will uncover all sorts of missed doses with the same patient through the use of the technique of "normalizing missed doses." I am reminded of the famous words of the social scientist Thomas Kuhn, "The answers you get depend upon the questions you ask."[5]

INTERVIEWING TIP #19:   Exploring Workplace Stigmatization

In the beginning of the chapter, I mentioned that the inconvenience of taking a medication at work can be problematic for some patients. In some instances, the boss of a facility has created a hostile environment toward patients with long-term illnesses. In other instances, patients with specific diseases, such as epilepsy, depression, and AIDS may be wary of sharing this information at the workplace, secondary to stigmatization issues in the culture. Because these concerns are universal in nature, I have found it useful to raise the issue of workplace stigmatization with my patients even when they do not raise it spontaneously. On occasion, I have been surprised by the intensity of the problem, an intensity that had clearly led to missed doses and, at times, had given the patient thoughts of stopping the medication altogether. The following simple question serves as a nice introduction to the topic:

"Are you having any problems with taking the pills at work?"

INTERVIEWING TIP #20:   Minimizing Workplace Stigmatization
                          with the "Vitamin Bottle Decoy"

Samir Tuma, a clinical associate professor of medicine at the University of Texas Medical School, offers a clever strategy for dealing with workplace stigmatization. He finds that the following advice is often greatly appreciated:

"I have found that there is a very simple way to deal with this problem. At home keep your medication in its standard bottle. But bring a couple of your pills to work in a tiny, but well-labeled empty "vitamin bottle." Then you can pull the bottle out anytime at lunch or where most appropriate, and, if anybody asks, just rave about how much benefit you've been getting from vitamin C or whatever vitamin you choose to rave about. No one will give it a second thought."

We have finished our exploration of the second belief set, cost, that patients use as they weigh the pros and cons of a medication. These costs can range from the traditional idea of financial burden to the less recognized idea of psychological inconvenience. As we have seen, just as Howard Brody stated at the beginning of the chapter, it is critical to uncover the patient's perceptions and how they define the problems. In the next chapter we will discover that perhaps the most important perception to uncover is a bit of a surprise. Sometimes patients, especially those destined to long-term use of medications, use the fact that they have to take a medication as the determining factor of how they define themselves. Their resulting definitions are seldom flattering. The result can be devastating for medication interest.

REFERENCES

1. Brody H. *The Healer's Power.* New Haven: Yale University Press; 1992:38–39.
2. Ellison JM. Enhancing adherence in the pharmacotherapy treatment relationship. In: Tasman A, Riba M, and Silk K, eds. *The Doctor-Patient Relationship in Pharmacotherapy.* New York, Guilford Press; 2000:84.
3. Steele DJ, Jackson TC, Gutmann MC. Have you been taking your pills? The adherence-monitoring sequence in the medical interview. *J Fam Pract* 1990;30(3):294–299.
4. Shea SC. *Psychiatric Interviewing: The Art of Understanding,* 2nd Ed. Philadelphia: WB Saunders; 1998:401–403.
5. Bayles D, Orland T. *Art & Fear.* Santa Barbara, CA: Capra Press, 1993:93.

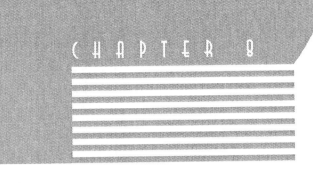

A Question of Meaning

"It is much more important to know what sort of patient has a disease than to know what sort of disease a patient has."[1]

Sir William Osler, MD

THE SOUL OF THE PILL

It is not so much that a pill has a soul. It is that each pill has an impact on the soul of those who take it. This impact is particularly prominent with patients who are destined to be on medications for many years, perhaps indefinitely. If you must reach for a pill bottle several times a day, over 700 times a year, tens of thousands of times over a lifetime, then that pill is going to assume a meaning to you, personally. The pill will become a symbol, and, for many patients, this meaning is translated into a question, "What does it say *about me* that I *have* to take this drug?"

Such a question moves the patient inexorably toward deeper questions concerned with meaning – who they are, and why do they have to take this drug that other people do not? For many patients these are disturbing questions with disturbing answers; for others graceful resolutions exist. The former patients stop their medications, and the latter patients stay on them.

This chapter has particular significance regarding patients suffering from severe and chronic illnesses, including multiple sclerosis, rheumatoid arthritis, epilepsy, cancer, schizophrenia, bipolar disorder, lupus erythematosus, renal failure, congestive heart failure, strokes, chronic pain syndromes, AIDS, and the list goes on and on. It is a list that none of us would like to be on, yet one that all of us know may await us someday.

The truth be told, these are diseases of fear, and the medications that help control and occasionally cure them assume a larger-than-life meaning to both the patient and the physician trying to comfort that patient. These strikingly high stakes are another reason that these medications cut directly to the substance of the patient's soul, and, for that matter, the soul of the doctor.

As we have seen while we examined the issues of efficacy and cost, the patient's perceptions shape the only viable reality with regards to medication interest. As Osler said, it is critical to understand what type of patient has a disease, because it is the uniqueness of the patients that will determine the uniqueness of these perceptions. Ultimately, to understand our patients, we must also understand, not only what they think about their diseases, but also what they think about the medications that they are now forced to take because of their diseases.

Peter Conrad's article, *The Meaning of Medications: Another Look at Compliance*[2] provides a wonderful introduction into this highly private world. In the following pages we will often refer to it.

Over the years, I have come to realize that it is the third set of beliefs, the meaning of the medication to the patients themselves, that is often the major determinant of long-term medication interest. In particular, an understanding of this set of beliefs is of particular value in explaining the many instances in which a patient suddenly stops an extremely important medication for what appears to be no good reason.

In such situations of puzzling medication discontinuance we often find that, concerning the first belief set, the patients feel that the symptom relief brought by the medication outweighs its side effects. Concerning the second belief set, these patients also view the benefits as outweighing both the financial costs and their costs to convenience. Yet these same patients stop the medications anyway (in which case the results are often catastrophic), the patient with a stable bipolar disorder goes into a series of manic rages, the MS patient returns to the confines of the wheelchair, and the AIDS patient plummets into a death spiral. Everyone is puzzled.

This chapter tries to unravel that puzzle. In the process, it may help us to recognize why these sudden drops in medication interest occur, and perhaps, through this knowledge decrease the likelihood that they have to happen. To unravel this puzzle, we will now turn to the internal world of our patients coping with AIDS.

AIDS: The Hidden Loss

The list of losses that a patient with AIDS may face is staggering: loss of functioning, loss of livelihood, loss of financial security, loss of friends due to stigmatization, loss of a sense of well-being secondary to symptoms, and, not least in nature, potential loss of life. These losses are so dramatic that they often overshadow another much more subtle but intensely painful loss. It is a hidden loss that most of our AIDS patients and, indeed, most of our patients with severe and chronic illnesses must deal with on a moment-by-moment basis.

The loss stems from the fact that, from the moment we turn to one of our patients and say, "I'm sorry to have to say that it looks like you have AIDS (or cancer or rheumatoid arthritis)," the lives of these patients will never be the same again. They immediately, in a matter of seconds, lose the ability to live life without thinking that they may soon lose that life or the ability to enjoy it. It is a haunting fear and a nagging enemy. In some respects, this hidden loss, the ability to not think about "being diseased," may be one of the greatest losses of all.

An understanding of this loss and its immense ramifications pulls us into the heart of our discussion concerning the meaning of medications and the patient's soul. At first glance one might think that AIDS patients would have minimal problems with taking their medications because the cost of not taking the medications, that is, death, is so striking. But medication interest is sometimes quite problematic with AIDS patients.

Part of this low medication interest is logical and easily recognized by all. It has to do with the second belief system from our last chapter, cost, both cost of the medications themselves and the incredible inconvenience of having to take 14 or so medications, some of which look like horse pills, three or four times a day. Some of these patients are literally gagging down these medications.

The other part of the problem stems directly from the hidden cost that we have been discussing and its impact on the meaning of the medications to the patient. For some patients with AIDS, these medications come to symbolize hope. They are viewed as "god-sends." These patients have high medication interest and will tolerate surprisingly severe degrees of both side effects and inconvenience.

On the other side of the continuum we find a different set of AIDS patients. These patients are coping with the constant awareness of their disease and the appalling shadow that this awareness casts on their ability to simply "enjoy life" without fear and worry. Some of these AIDS patients would figuratively "give their right arms" to be able to live a three month period again, during which time they would have absolutely no idea that they had AIDS – to savor once more the immense luxury of living life without this lingering shadow.

For these patients the pills and their pill bottles may come to symbolize not hope but despair. Three or four times every day, just as they were about to lose awareness of their illnesses, they must reach for these bottles to be reminded of it. Our medications, without any intention on our parts, have come to symbolize not that there is help for their disease but that they are "diseased."

The medications have become constant reminders that life can never be the same again. For some of these patients – and I feel it is a very human and very normal response indeed – it all just becomes too much. They think, "I can't put up with this anymore. I just don't give a damn." Then they skip some doses or even stop them altogether.

Described here is a prime example of how a patient's perception of a medication can help define that patient's perception of himself or herself. What, at first glance, had appeared as a puzzling discontinuance of medication, at second glance, makes sense. The discontinuance of the medication is a protective response for a person who is striving to get away from the self-perception that "I am diseased."

INTERVIEWING TIP #21:   Changing "Tapes"

I want to return for a moment to an interviewing technique described in Chapter 3, that was provided by a pulmonologist, Ed Hamaty, regarding motivating patients via their desire to "be there" for their families. If you will recall he had suggested that helping patients to create a phrase to repeat when reaching for their medications, such as, "This is for my granddaughter," could be powerfully motivating.

Hamaty goes on to provide an even more sophisticated method of conceptualizing these affirmations, that goes far beyond their use as family motivators. He suggests that patients often unknowingly adapt some of the demoralizing thoughts described previously into scripts that are automatically played with every dosage. He first noticed this counterproductive process with his AIDS patients but soon found the problem to be ubiquitous across many chronic diseases. As taking the pills becomes more psychologically painful, patients begin to anticipate the unpleasantness of the upcoming pill taking. In essence, they begin to "play a tape" that sounds something like, "Oh God, not this again" or "I'm so sick of being sick." Hamaty suggests that we can work with these patients to create positive affirmations designed to replace their naturally arising negative ones. The patient's demoralizing tape can thus be rerecorded into something much more comforting and inspiring for use as the patient reaches for his or her medications.

Picture a patient fighting AIDS, who feels a certain pride in his or her efforts against the AIDS virus, despite the fact that he or she is slowly becoming demoralized. For such a patient, the following two-word affirmation – "Take that!" – directed toward the AIDS virus itself may function almost like a personal act of releasing defiance.

To be maximally effective, each aphorism must be individually generated by the patient and have unique meaning to that patient. For instance, if the patient is suffering from intractable pain as he takes his pain medication, the patient might say, directed toward the pain, "Not today you don't."

The creation of such affirmations can be effective with patients dealing with psychiatric disorders as well. For example, many of my younger patients with OCD find it re-affirming to say something like the following: "This one is for you OCD, I'm gonna kick your butt today." Such affirmations externalize the disease so that the patient does not view himself or herself as the problem while focusing the patient on his or her ability to control the OCD symptoms, frequently using cognitive behavioral therapy techniques as well.

We can see that there are many things we can try to do to help with intense demoralization, from checking to see whether a major depression is on board that may respond to antidepressants, to rallying the patient's support systems, to changing the patient's demoralizing "tape." But even our best efforts do not change the fact that there is ample reason to be demoralized by the presence of a fatal or lingering illness. The acceptance of such a momentous loss is never an easy path for anyone, patient or physician. Nor can it be.

This inescapable dilemma of both past and modern medicine – that our medications are not always able to stop death – reminds us of a very important point from Chapter 1, a point pertaining to the role of the therapeutic alliance that bears repeating now: "The remainder of this book is an effort to show some of the concrete techniques that can help prescribing clinicians effectively do their part to define this potentially powerful alliance, the alliance that helps us to heal when healing is possible and to comfort when it is not."

It reminds us that one of the most important functions that we serve as physicians is to be there not only when we are offering hope for cure, but also when we are communicating that no such hope exists. Such moments of exquisite anguish, and their aftermath, may very well be the moments in which it is most important for us to be there for our patients.

As Thomas Gordon and W. Sterling Edwards point out in their sensitive and insightful book, *Making the Patient Your Partner*, one of the greatest fears that a patient with a fatal illness has is that once the physician cannot offer a cure, the physician will disappear.[3] They go on to add that simple comments such as, "Don't worry, despite the bad news, I have no intention of abandoning you. I'll see you as often as necessary and we'll fight this thing together" can be extraordinarily reassuring to patients.

It is over the effectiveness or ultimate impotence of our medications that these moments are most apt to arise, hence the importance of their discussion in this book. It is an opportune time to remember that it is our ability to convey our caring that is often the cornerstone of our healing and our ability to comfort. It also reminds us that, when our patients or their family members find themselves crying as they face the loss of hope for a cure, the greatest gift we have to offer is often simply our own tears.

Transforming Damaging Myths and the Bite of Cultural Stigmatization

Bearing a chronic illness requires patients to carry the weight of two crosses. They must not only bear the weight that their illnesses bring to them but also the weight that other people foster upon them for having those illnesses. Stigmatization can occur across a wide range of diseases, including juvenile onset diabetes, seizure disorders, AIDS, cancer, and, of course, mental illnesses. These latter illnesses (mental illnesses) may very well stand as the "granddaddy's of stigmatization." As such, gathering an understanding of the impact of stigmatization with these diseases may help us to better understand how to transform the stigmatization that can be found in many other diseases.

The purpose of this book is not to explore the complex role and nuances of the stigmatization of those who have mental illnesses. The purpose is to uncover the role of the stigmatization of the medications used to treat these illnesses. As we saw earlier, the negative views that patients have toward their medications is often insidiously transformed into a negative view of themselves. This negativity can drop the bottom out of medication interest. This damaging phenomenon is well worth our attention, because we can frequently transform it through the use of sound interviewing technique.

The stigmatization of psychiatric medications, and, consequently, of oneself for needing them, is not solely the domain of major psychiatric disorders, such as schizophrenia and bipolar disorder. It can also be seen with much milder forms of mental disorder, the types that are seen in the offices of both psychiatrists and primary care physicians on a daily basis.

For instance, a high functioning woman who was the manager of a medical office and was suffering from a moderately severe depression poignantly described her feelings of stigmatization as follows:

"Please don't get me wrong. I really appreciate how much this medication has helped me. But if I'm honest with both you and myself, every time I reach for it, I feel as if I am defective. I just do. I don't know why."

Experiencing such a negative feeling about oneself once, and sometimes multiple times, every day, as one uncaps his or her pill bottle, is no small matter. Returning to our metaphor of the patient having an internal committee that is voting "yea" or "nay" on the issue of staying on a medication, it is easy enough to guess this member's vote. From this point of view, considering stopping the medication is logical; taking the medication is causing psychological damage at least once or twice every day. Such psychological damage is a very real and very bad side effect.

Imagine the negative consequences of this stigma for patients coping with schizophrenia or bipolar disorder. Despite my team's best efforts to destigmatize these illnesses for these patients, some of them became convinced that they were the problem, not the illness. When these patient's reached for their medications, they were often experiencing profoundly disturbing thoughts, such as, "They all think I'm crazy. Maybe I am after all. Maybe I'm just worthless. The only way I can function is if they drug me." Needless to say, this type of brutal self-denigration is a significant "con" to taking any medication. It would not be illogical for a patient experiencing this type of daily battering to consider discontinuing his or her medication. It is common sense.

Especially with psychiatric medications, but also with medications for nonpsychiatric disorders, two widely held myths predispose patients toward such self-denigrations. Let us look at what these myths are and some of the effective strategies for dismantling them.

INTERVIEWING TIP #22:   Dismantling the "Addiction Myth"

Especially with regards to antidepressants, the myth that these medications are addictive is so prevalent in our culture, that if the topic is not spontaneously raised by the patient, I will raise it myself as follows:

"There is a common misconception about antidepressants, that I just wanted to address with you, because you may run in to it. Many people quite naturally, and you might have some of these concerns yourself, are worried that these medications are addictive. First of all, I would always tell you if a medication I was giving you was addictive or not. Second, these medications simply are not.

"They do not make you high. I have never seen anyone in my entire career crave them; in fact, drug addicts get mad at me if I prescribe them, because they want addictive drugs instead.

"Let me explain exactly how they work. All of our brain cells depend upon small molecules that function as messengers from one cell to the next. These messenger molecules are called *neurotransmitters*. We will simply call them *messengers*.

"With depression you may have low amounts of the messengers called *serotonin* or *norepinephrine*. It is exactly like diabetes, where the patient's pancreas is low on making insulin. The appropriate treatment for diabetes is to give the patient insulin so it gets back to a normal level. Insulin is not an addictive medication even though the patient must take it every day. We are simply getting the person's insulin level back to normal.

"In depression the brain may be low on serotonin, and so we give the patient a medication that raises the serotonin level back to normal. Serotonin is not addictive, no more than insulin is. Both insulin and serotonin are naturally in your body but low in diabetes and depression."

I then continue with education on how the medications work, and I may make drawings of the synapse for patients or refer to pre-made patient educational aids that they can take home.

When flexibly modified for both the patient's intellectual functioning and the patient's interest in hearing the information, interviewing techniques, such as "dismantling the addiction myth," are quite useful in undercutting the addiction myth before it can wreak havoc on medication interest.

Some of the shorter-acting SSRIs may, if they are discontinued abruptly, have physiological effects. When using such medications, I address this issue as follows:

"By the way, you may have heard that if you suddenly stop some antidepressants you can get some unwanted side effects, sometimes called the *withdrawal syndrome*. This is because your body has made some small adjustments to the medication over the long term. It is not the same as being addicted to a drug. There is no psychological craving for these meds. Moreover, the withdrawal syndrome does not happen if you taper off the medication slowly, which we always would, and I myself have seldom seen problems with this process. Let me explain what symptoms you might get if you suddenly stopped the medication."

I then proceed to alert the patient to the possible problems that could be encountered. I find once again that patients are quite comfortable with such a matter-of-fact approach.

INTERVIEWING TIP #23:   Dismantling "the Crutch Myth"

A second myth, that the medication is a crutch, is so common with antidepressants that I address it directly after dismantling the addiction myth as follows:

> "There is another common misconception that these medications are crutches, that somehow you should be able to cope with depression without medications. But if your brain is not making enough serotonin, it simply isn't making enough serotonin, and you can't just 'will it' to make more, any more than a person with diabetes can will their pancreas to make more insulin. We would never tell a person with diabetes that their insulin is a crutch because it isn't. We are simply getting their insulin back to the normal level that everyone else has.
>
> "It is exactly the same with your depression. Your brain is not making enough serotonin, and we are just going to get your serotonin back to the normal level that everybody else has. It isn't a crutch. It is getting your serotonin level back to normal, so that you then have a fair chance to effectively cope with your stresses. Don't let anyone tell you it is a crutch, because it is simply not true."

I have had good luck with this approach or variations of it. Give it a try and see what you think.

The small amount of time these two approaches require – and although it is a relatively small amount of time it is not an insignificant amount when you only have seven to fifteen minutes with a patient – can pay off in a big way in increasing medication interest. Without such proactive comments, many patients will have stopped their antidepressants by the next visit, necessitating the time-consuming process of introducing yet another new medication. Furthermore, if, following the medication discontinuation, the patient's depression worsens it may, ultimately, require more frequent appointments or even hospitalizations.

In such instances, these few comments, that indeed cost us a few minutes, may save many hours of clinical time as well as thousands of dollars if hospitalization had resulted. The proactive use of these two simple interviewing techniques, dismantling the addiction myth and dismantling the crutch myth, is a win-win-win situation (saves the patient from suffering, saves the physician time, saves the system money).

INTERVIEWING TIP #24:   Getting a Read on the Patient's Medication Grapevine

Concerning familiarity with medications, the culture of today is a far cry from the culture of the early 1980s, when I first trained in medicine. Today, patients are much more informed about medication choices. The "medication grapevine" is vastly improved. In my opinion, for the most part, this turn of events is a very good one, but there are a few downsides as well. Popular media and the Web sometimes contribute to the stigmatization problem by presenting false and unwarranted biases against medications that can lower medication interest sometimes precipitously. While I was providing a workshop in Tampa, Florida, Bruce Edson, a primary care physician, offered a nice tip for uncovering such potentially damaging misconceptions in his daily practice. Edson asks:

> "Sometimes this medication can help with problems like you are having. Have you heard anything good or bad – from the Internet, magazines, radio, or television – about this medication?"

By specifically mentioning various channels of cultural bias (i.e., "Internet, magazines, radio, or television"), I believe the clinician increases the likelihood that the patient will provide the whole scoop from the grapevine.

Another workshop participant, Lucius Ripley, suggests following up this strategy by providing patients with specific Web sites that are objective and demonstrate neither a bias for nor against the medication in question (such as might be provided by NIH or NIMH). Armed first with this factual knowledge, if the patient surfs the Web and comes upon negative Web sites and antimedicine rhetoric, the patient will be better armed to view such information objectively. In addition, having first visited the unbiased Web sites suggested by the clinician, it is much more likely that the patient will subsequently feel comfortable going to the Web sites provided by pharmaceutical companies, where they can find much valuable information.

THE CURIOUS PARADOX OF SUCCESS: WHY PATIENTS "TEST"

Perhaps one of the most frustrating phenomena for psychiatrists occurs when patients, devastated by bipolar disorder who finally achieve freedom from their symptoms, suddenly choose to stop their mood stabilizers and antipsychotics. Soon the lives of these patients are again in shambles, and the whole vicious cycle has restarted.

Some of these patients stop the medications because the mania begins to break-through their current dosage. Mania, by its very nature makes people feel powerful and invulnerable, so it is only natural that these patients are prompted, by the disease process itself, to stop their medications. This type of patient is worrisome, but their relapse is both understandable, and, perhaps, even predictable.

But there are other patients with bipolar disorder in complete remission, who are intelligent, motivated for health, psychologically intact, well aware of the potential risks, and are even vocal

proponents of the usefulness of medications, who suddenly stop
their medications and rapidly deteriorate. These patients are often
a puzzlement and a frustration for psychiatrists, case managers,
family members, colleagues, and even themselves.

For me, the insight into these patients and their self-induced
relapses, came not from my own clinical work, but once again
from the writings of Peter Conrad and his work with patients
with epilepsy. Let us see what Conrad uncovered.

First, Conrad discovered that patients who had their epilepsy
in excellent control would sometimes do exactly what my patients
with bipolar disorder would do: abruptly stop their medications.
Let us hear why this occurred from one of Conrad's patients
herself:

> "When I was young I would try not to take it . . . I'd take it for
> a while and think, 'Well, I don't need it anymore,' so I would
> not take it for, deliberately, just to see if I could do without. And
> then (in a few days) I'd start takin' it again, because I'd start
> passin' out . . . I will still try that now, when my husband is out
> of town . . . I just think, maybe I'm still gonna grow out of it or
> something."

Conrad's patient sheds a brilliant light upon the curious
paradox that unfolds when medications are effective in relieving symptoms. Indeed, if a medication removes all symptoms –
whether in bipolar disorder or a seizure disorder – the paradox
is at its maximum. Simply stated, if a medication successfully
removes all symptoms, it removes any ability for the patient to
know whether or not the disease is still active.

Some psychiatric diseases, such as major depressive disorder,
sometimes do go completely away and never return. With such
diseases, patients are in a bind. They may have to decide to stay
on a medication for the rest of their lives, although they may not
need it.

When medications completely relieve symptoms, paradoxically, the problem with the *meaning* of the medication is that patients

no longer know what it means. They no longer know what they really have and, indirectly, it can feel as if they do not know who they really are. Conrad summarizes far better than I can, what intelligent patients with epilepsy will face if their medications remove all symptoms:

"But how can one know that a period without seizures is a result of medication or spontaneous remission of the disorder? How long can one go without medication? How 'bad' is this case of epilepsy? How can one know if epilepsy is 'getting better' while still taking medication? Usually, after a period without or with only a few seizures, many reduced or stopped their medicine altogether to test for themselves whether or not epilepsy was 'still' there."

With my bipolar patients, the discontinuance of their medications is no longer a mystery or a puzzlement. It makes good sense. It is not comfortable or natural to not know what is going on inside one's body. The urge to "test" is not the hallmark of "opposition" or "lack of insight." It is the attempt to gain insight.

INTERVIEWING TIP #25:   Testing the Waters

When I have a patient in good remission, I will periodically ask something along this order:

"Jim, you've been doing great on your medications now for over a year. It's wonderful that you have your bipolar disorder (substitute whatever illness the patient is dealing with) in excellent control. Some of my patients tell me that after awhile, they get curious about whether or not they still have the bipolar disorder or even need the medications. I think that is a natural curiosity. Do you ever have thoughts like that?"

Depending upon what the patient says, one can gain insight as to whether the patient's committee is getting ready to vote for a "med-free trial." Sometimes the physician can convince the patient's committee that such a trial is not advisable. Such proactive questioning by the physician can prevent a tragedy and, in some instances, where suicidal ideation is a common aspect of relapse, even save a life.

I should add one other note. In rare and carefully screened patients (i.e., patients where processes such as suicide and violence are not part of the patient's symptom history), I have found that if a patient is absolutely determined to stop a medication, it is sometimes better that I first make the suggestion to do so myself. More specifically, I suggest that we taper the medication under carefully controlled circumstances, and with support systems well alerted. In contrast to the frequently deep tailspins that patients experience when they secretly and abruptly stop all their medications, I have found that, in some instances, such controlled tapers allow the treatment team to halt the decompensation much earlier and to restabilize the patient with much smaller doses.

I only do this type of taper if the patient agrees to carefully look for early warning symptoms of relapse and to restart the medication, if necessary, and the patient agrees to view it as a legitimate test to see whether the disease is still present. If relapse occurs, it is not uncommon for such patients to gain insight into the need for their medication.

For example, I had one patient, with schizo-affective disorder, who had resisted medications for years and had consistently been in and out of hospitals several times every year. He hated being in the hospital but always ended up creating long hospitalizations for himself by stopping his medications secretly and abruptly. Eventually, he agreed to a controlled taper. After three such controlled trials, and resulting brief hospitalizations, he walked into my office and said, "You know what, Dr. Shea, I guess I really need this shit!"

He has continued on his medications from that day onward. At a later point, he added, "I still don't think I have this schizo-whatever thing. But I am sick of landing in the hospital, and I do get wired up without my lithium."

THE MEANING OF THE MEDICATIONS OUTSIDE THE PATIENT'S HEAD:
"THE K STREET LOBBY"

In this chapter we have been looking at how patients use the personal meaning of their medications as a means of weighing the pros and cons, the third step of the Choice Triad. We have seen that, in addition to weighing their symptom relief versus their side effects and their benefits versus their costs (both financially and with regards to convenience), patients also put a high premium upon the meaning of their medications. The symbolic message attached to the need to take a medication either makes patients feel better or worse about themselves.

This symbolic meaning often explains unexpected drops in medication interest, even to the point of discontinuance. As we have explored the nuances of this meaning, we have seen that these "unexplainable" drops in medication interest are actually quite explainable and merely represent human beings trying to take some control over what often appears uncontrollable.

In essence, it really is as if the patient held within his or her head a multitude of opinions or voices regarding each medication and its meaning. Some of the voices are for the medication and some against it. But one more set of voices remain from whom we have yet to hear, but these voices are outside the patient's head: the lobbyists so to speak. Like the lobbyists on K Street in Washington, DC, who aggressively push their agenda, many people associated with the patient will aggressively express opinions as to whether it is a good idea or a bad idea to take a medication. Unfortunately, many patients translate this opinion into a reflection of their self image as to whether they are good people or bad people, smart people or dumb people, for having chosen "to be on meds."

The simple truth is that we don't so much prescribe for a single patient as we prescribe for family units. The opinions of the patient's nuclear family, spouses/partners, parents, and siblings sometimes sway the patient the most, even more than our opinions as physicians. And their "extended families," their peers, fellow patients at the community mental health center, and friends, also have a powerful lobbying status. Many a patient has stopped a medication because of the horror stories that a friend has animatedly related to them about the medication.

Following our basic principle (we want to hear the vote of the committee inside our offices), it becomes important to find out how these lobbyists are trying to sway the vote. Naturally, it is best to ask them directly. But, oftentimes, constraints and practicality make such inquiries not feasible. Fortunately, most patients are more than willing to fill us in on the opinions of their social supports, if we know what questions to ask.

INTERVIEWING TIP #26:   Probing for Resistance from the
                        Patient's Spouse/Partner

In our culture many strong biases exist against medications, especially psychiatric medications. If our patient's significant other has one of these biases, it can be deadly to medication interest. I have found the following question to be useful in uncovering such biases: "How do you think your spouse (partner) will feel about your starting on an antidepressant?"

A not uncommon reply is, "To tell you the truth, Charlie doesn't really believe in this kind of thing." Depending upon the methods by which Charlie expresses this opinion – ranging from mild discouragement to abusive anger – we may have uncovered a critical roadblock to medication interest. Also of importance is to remember that the patient's spouse/partner may also have strong opinions about medications used to treat nonpsychiatric disorders, including medications for seizure control, cancer, hypertension, diabetes, and erectile dysfunction as well as birth control pills and hormone replacements.

Sometimes, when the patient indicates that there may be considerable resistance from a spouse/partner, it is best to not begin the medication immediately but to suggest that the significant other accompany the patient next time. Such face-to-face meetings with the patient's spouse/partner allow us to both better assess the potential roadblock and, not uncommonly, offer us a chance to transform it. In the last analysis, few better ways exist to change a committee's negative vote than to meet with the key lobbyists who are equally intent on procuring this vote. Once again, the extra time it takes to meet with our patient's spouse/partner can save us hours of time wasted in future appointments mandated by a patient whose depression or seizure disorder is out of control.

INTERVIEWING TIP #27:   Anticipating Friends' Opinions on
                                          Medications

Once again, friends can play the determining influence on medication interest for "the good" or "the bad." On the good side of the continuum, imagine the powerful boost to medication interest if a friend comments, "Oh my gosh, that's the same drug I used for my depression. It's great. I'm not kidding you; it saved my life."

Contrast this boost to the damage resulting at the other end of the continuum, "Oh my God! Don't you dare take that horrible thing. I tried it once and it was horrendous. You will feel like a zombie. I'm not kidding . . . (pause) . . . you know, I heard that some people are killing people on that stuff." We might as well have asked the patient to just drop off that prescription in the trash can as he or she walked out our office door.

As time permits, you may find the following question to be invaluable: "Do you have any friends who have taken this medication, and, if so, what did they think of it?"

As intimated earlier, community mental health centers are cultures unto themselves, with a robust grapevine among patients. (Note that at some centers some patients may prefer being called *consumers* or *clients,* yet another example of the unique culture within each center.) The reputation of certain medications can be positive or negative with patients, and they will share their opinions often and strongly with each other. In this regard, I have found the following variant of the previous question also useful to ask: "Have you heard anything good or bad about this medication from other patients (consumers/clients)?"

INTERVIEWING TIP #28:   Looking for Bad Associations That A
                        Teenager May Have with a Medication

For most kids and teenagers, considerable stigma still exist with taking medications, from asthma medications to attention deficit medications. Few students are comfortable pulling an inhaler out before gym class or trotting off to the school nurse to get a pill. Consequently, it is useful to ask younger patients what it is like to be taking a medication at school or on the playground.

On the other hand, a pediatrician, who treats many children with hyperactivity, told me that he has noticed a change in attitude in a small number of kids over the past decade regarding their psychiatric medications. Some kids are now talking about them a lot. "I'm taking this." "I'm taking that." "I'm on Ritalin." "I'm selling Ritalin." You name it, it comes out of their mouths. For a small number of students, especially those students in middle or high school, being on a psychiatric medication has become an "in thing."

Consequently, it is possible that the teenager you are prescribing for has already heard something at school about the medication that you are about to prescribe. As with adults, that "something" might not be too good. The following question can ferret out this roadblock to medication interest quite easily: "Do you have any friends or know of anyone at school who has taken this medication?"

The subsequent exchange may go something like this:

Patient: Yea . . . (*The student starts squirming in his or her seat.*) . . .
        Jimmy Wilson.
Physician: Who is Jimmy Wilson?
Patient: (*Further squirming.*) He's the biggest geek in the school,
        Doc. I'm not kidding you. Geek city.

If so, at such moments the astute clinician has the choice of proceeding, "Well, if you just take this medication that I'm offering you, you too can become a total geek in just under a month" or "Well, perhaps we can find a medication that works in a similar fashion but which you might be more comfortable with. How does that sound to you?" It doesn't take a rocket scientist to figure out the more effective path for increasing medication interest. But the choice of paths would not have been known, unless the clinician had asked the above question.

INTERVIEWING TIP #29:   Selective Use of Clinician
                          "Self-Transparency"

As we wrap up our survey of interviewing techniques for use in navigating the tricky waters of lobbyists and their influences, it is useful to remember an important lobbyist not yet mentioned – us. Patients often have a high regard for our opinions, which leads us to the topic of selective "self-transparency." If the clinician feels comfortable with self-transparency and is selective when to use it, sharing something about oneself can be useful in an effort to destigmatize a medication.

A workshop participant of mine, Aida Li, has found self-transparency to be occasionally useful in destigmatizing. For instance, if the patient appears frightened about a medication, such as an asthma medication or a medication for congestive heart failure, she might comment, if true: "You know, my mother is on this medication and thinks it is just great."

At times it can be useful to share one's own experience:

"You know, Jim, I've been on this same medication for my high blood pressure for years, and it has been a super med for me. My blood pressure has been great and any side effects went away quickly."

When a patient hears that the prescribing clinician is using the same medication, it is hard to imagine a more credible endorsement.

We have now completed our discussion of the importance of

the meaning of the medication to influence medication interest. The patient may view the symbolic meaning of the medication as a powerful pro or as a powerful con. In either case, an exploration of this meaning is one of the major pathways to understanding what "sort of patient has a disease," as Sir William Osler suggested at the beginning of the chapter.

Furthermore, with the last four chapters, we have also completed our exploration of the individual nuances that impact on how each patient navigates the third step of the Choice Triad: weighing the pros and cons. From the perspective of our metaphor, we have uncovered various interviewing techniques that make it more likely that the patient's committee will vote inside our offices not outside them. This ability to help our patients clearly and openly share their views on the pros and cons of their medications is, in my opinion, one of the most important sets of skills that a physician can develop. These skills are at the very heart of enhancing medication interest.

As we near the end of our book, it is enlightening to return once again to the basic principles of the medication interest model, because there is still much that they have to offer now that we are more comfortable with their use.

REFERENCES

1. Osler W. Website of the Global Family Doctor at www.globalfamilydoctor. com/LighterSide/QuotableQuotes.asp (5/29/06).
2. Conrad P. The meaning of medications: another look at compliance. *Soc Sci Med* 1985;20(1):29–37.
3. Gordon T, Edwards WS. *Making the Patient Your Partner.* Westport, CT: Auburn House, 1997.

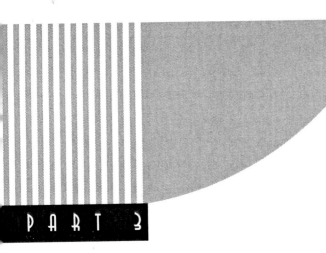

PART 3

Helping Patients
Make the Right
Choice:
**Finding
Solutions**

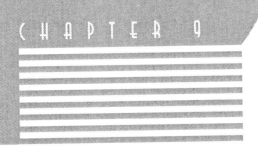

CHAPTER 9

Medication Interest Redux – Caring for the Patient

"One of the essential qualities of the clinician is interest in humanity, for the secret of the care of the patient is in caring for the patient."[1]

Francis Peabody, MD

Journal of the American Medical Association

(88th Volume, 1927)

P
eabody's quotation has always been one of my favorites. It seems to embody the very essence of our work, and it is as fresh today as it was seven decades ago. The quotation also has a not-so-small connection with the topic of our book – medication interest. We have already seen that it is from the introduction, discussion, and negotiation of medications that much of the physician/patient alliance evolves and shapes itself. In many respects, a patient will determine just how much the physician "cares" by the words with which that physician introduces medications and discusses side-effect. In essence, this book has been a primer of how to take Peabody's poignant sentiment and transform it into clinical practice.

As we come to the end of our book, it is a good time to review the fundamentals of the medication interest model, which, as we said before is both a philosophy of how to talk with patients about their medications and a model of possible ways to do so. The following is a summary of the key elements of the philosophy discussed, so far. The summary will help us to more clearly see where we have been. It will also point the direction that we must go in our final chapter, if we want to bring Peabody's words to life in the hectic exam rooms of a primary care clinic or in the busy offices of a community mental health center.

THE CORE PRINCIPLES OF THE "MEDICATION INTEREST" PHILOSOPHY

1. The introduction, discussion, and negotiation of medication use is one of the primary interactions from which the physician/patient alliance defines itself.
2. The less opposition a patient feels coming from the prescriber, the more open the patient will be to the prescriber's medication recommendations.
3. The majority of patients who choose to refuse medications, change how they are taken, or stop them altogether are not being oppositional but are making the wisest choices that they can, using the beliefs that they currently hold.
4. The prescriber's job, as an educator, is to uncover these beliefs, reinforce those that are correct, correct those that are false, and provide new information that can be of immediate use to the patient.
5. While providing this education on medications, the prescriber should consciously choose words that create a sensation of "going with" the patient while minimizing feelings of "going against" the patient's perspective.
6. Within the fields of medicine and psychiatry, a concerted effort should be made to discover interviewing techniques, for use while discussing medications, that foster this feeling of "going with" the patient.

7. Understanding how patients choose medications is essential for developing such interviewing techniques.
8. Patients choose to take a medication if they navigate the following three processes, known as the Choice Triad:
    I. The patient believes something is wrong.
    II. The patient is motivated to use a medication to do something about it.
    III. The patient is convinced that the pros of the medication outweigh the cons.
9. Patients weigh the pros and cons by looking at three belief sets, generated from three corresponding questions. These belief sets and their corresponding questions are as follows:
    I. Efficacy (Does this drug make me feel better?)
    II. Cost (Is it worth it to me to take this drug?)
    III. Meaning (What does it say about me that I have to take this drug?)
10. An understanding of how patients choose medications allows us to develop specific interviewing techniques that can enhance medication interest.
11. Once developed, these interviewing techniques should be concretely operationalized and behaviorally defined.
12. Once these techniques have been operationalized and defined, they should be named.
13. Once operationalized, defined, and named, these interviewing techniques can be taught, and the clinician's competence to perform them tested.
14. Once operationalized, defined, and named, these interviewing techniques become amenable to empirical study.
15. From such empirical studies weak techniques can be deleted, effective techniques refined, and new techniques developed.
16. Gradual progress can be made in developing evidence-based interviewing strategies that tend to increase our patient's interest in starting medications and staying on them.

In this book we have come a long way toward developing this model. In our closing chapter we return to the very heart of the model, as reflected in the first six principles. In these opening principles we see a strong emphasis on avoiding oppositional feelings toward the patient as we create a collaborative sensation of "going with" the patient. Only then do we become true partners with the patient. As we close, we will focus upon this element of the medication interest model, discovering that it is not only the heart of the model, but also the gateway through which Peabody's sense of caring flows.

MEDICATION INTEREST AND THE FIRST APPOINTMENT: A SECOND GLANCE

We have discussed the first appointment at length, but a second glance may yield fresh perspectives and some new interviewing techniques. One of the first keys to fostering a collaborative sensation, as opposed to an oppositional one, is to make sure that the physician knows exactly with what the patient wants help.

This idea might sound almost comically obvious, but there is a catch here. Physicians are frequently trained to treat diseases - congestive heart failure, diabetes, posttraumatic stress disorder - but patients usually want help with symptoms – "can't breathe," "feel weak," "have flashbacks." Right from the beginning, a potential disconnect exists between the physician's goals and the patient's goals. Knowing exactly what symptoms are most problematic for the patient is often invaluable, because our patients will often judge the success of our treatments, not through an abstract improvement in their diseases but through a concrete relief from their symptoms.

Sometimes my assumptions as to what symptoms must be most troubling to my patients are surprisingly inaccurate. I may have a patient with a severe depression and suicidal ideation, with whom I assume that the suicidal ideation is the most problematic symptom. To my surprise it is the inability to sleep that the patient relates as the most pressing problem, commenting, "I could cope with the suicidal stuff, if I just had some rest, but I'm completely drained, Dr. Shea, completely drained. I'd give my right arm if I could get a night's sleep."

INTERVIEWING TIP #30: Finding the Patient's Personal Target Symptoms

One of the more effective ways to see the world through our patients' eyes is to find out what they see as the most pressing symptom. One of the most convincing ways to subsequently show patients that we are "with them" is to do something about it. I have found questions, such as the following, to be effective at this undercover work:

1. "Mrs. Davis, of all of the different symptoms that you are getting from your heart problems, what are the ones that are most problematic for you?"
2. "Mrs. Davis, of all of your different heart symptoms, which are the ones you most want help with?"
3. "Mrs. Davis, if I had a magic pill, and I don't, but if I did, and it could completely take away just one of your heart symptoms, which one would you want me to get rid of?"

When through the use of such questions a physician and a patient can uncover which symptoms are most discouraging from the patient's standpoint and then agree to do something about those specific symptoms, patients truly feel that they are being heard, and, in fact, they are. Both ends of the stethoscope start liking each other a good deal more, and a team is being forged within minutes of the initial meeting.

Additionally, by asking directly which symptoms are most problematic from the patient's viewpoint, the physician obtains a clearer picture of "what sort of patient has a disease," as Sir William Osler emphasized in our last chapter. A symptom may mean something unique to each unique patient, and every patient is unique.

Such questioning can also point to which medication may be most effective from a given family of medications in relieving the symptom of most concern to the patient. With the depressed patient whom I described earlier, I am going to lean toward an antidepressant that will quickly help with sleep. At other times, the patient's self-identified target symptom may even suggest interventions other than pharmacological ones, for example, a relaxation tape for sleep induction.

Let us see this interviewing technique – finding the patient's personal target symptoms – as it creates a feeling of "going with" a patient in an initial meeting. Returning to Mrs. Davis, our CHF patient, imagine that in response to our attempt to elicit her personal target symptom she goes on to belatedly describe her intense embarrassment at not being able to get into her shoes because of the edema in her legs. Her shame has prevented her from going to shoe stores for several years, a shopping ritual she sorely misses, because she had always prided herself on having "nice, nothing fancy mind you, but nice shoes."

This tiny snapshot of "humanness" may seem, at first glance, mundane and unimportant, but it is not. It is exactly what Osler was looking for: "what sort of patient has a disease." It may, in its own unassuming way, hold the key to creating a powerful and lasting alliance with Mrs. Davis, because if we can find a medicine, such as a diuretic, that rapidly takes away her edema, we have found a medicine that Mrs. Davis is probably going to want to stay on. More importantly, Mrs. Davis has found a doctor that she is probably going to want to keep.

INTERVIEWING TIP #31:   Eliciting the Patient's Views on
                          Current Medications

Many of the patients that we are seeing for an initial H&P or for an initial psychiatric assessment, walk in the door with a bunch of medications already on board. Some patients have a preconceived notion that all doctors like all medications, and that the role of the physician is to make sure the patient stays on his or her meds. Naturally, such a preconception predisposes to the creation of an oppositional alliance.

A workshop participant at one of my Arizona workshops shared some questions that are useful for undercutting such a malproductive process before it can even raise its head. The questions assume the possibility that the current medications may or may not be totally pleasing to the patient, establishing the new physician's genuine interest in the patient's end of the stethoscope:

1. What is your understanding of the purpose of each of your medications?
2. Do they seem to help?
3. Do some help better than others?
4. Do you like your medications?
5. Were you interested in making any changes in any of them?
6. Do you think that you need to be on medications?
7. Have you ever thought of alternative treatments in addition to your medications or perhaps instead of them?

These questions also shed light on various useful bits of information, including patients' intelligence, patients' memory retention, patients' ability to express themselves, patients' ability to effectively assert their viewpoints. Patients' answers may also provide indirect information on the quality of the previous prescriber/patient alliance and the quality of previous education regarding medications. For a small number of questions, the previously described packet goes a long way toward fostering a nonoppositional partnership, while yielding surprisingly useful information.

INTERVIEWING TIP #32:   Eliciting Children's Views on
                        Their Medications

A social worker, Kay McAuliffe, pointed out to me that with children under ten, it is still important to uncover their personal views (as opposed to relying solely on their parents' views) as to "what this med business is all about." Medications can be extraordinarily confusing to kids and they may develop untrue and potentially worrisome distortions about their medications. She further points out that, although the clinician is basically covering the same material as with adults, there are some subtle changes in the wording that can make the inquiries more kid-friendly and effective at getting a child's true opinions. Such questions include:

1. "Why do you think you are taking this pill?"
2. "How is it supposed to help you?"
3. "Do you want to be taking it?"

The above two sets of questions suggest an intriguing point regarding patient apprehensions about medications when meeting us for the first time; it is a point that is often overlooked. For some patients the fear is not only that we are about to start a new medication. They also fear that we are about to stop an old one. To put it bluntly, the patient and family members are concerned that we are about "to monkey with the meds."

INTERVIEWING TIP #33:   Reassuring Family Members that No
                         Hasty Decisions are About to Be Made

Especially with psychiatric patients with severe and chronic disorders, such as schizophrenia, schizo-affective disorder, and bipolar disorders, the pain of the family members is truly beyond words. These diseases rape the souls of their children, torture them incessantly for years, and pit family member against family member.

Undoubtedly, numerous medication combinations and cocktails have been used, some effective, some ineffective, and some worse than the disease itself. Once a combination has been found that provides even a modicum of relief for the patient, family members are deeply grateful.

As one can well imagine, after years of failed treatment comɔinations, these family members, and often the patients as well, are terrified that the "new Doc" is going to change something and "screw up" everything. Sometimes they do. The family's fear, that a major medication change is imminent, can rise to almost panic proportions, especially if they have seen previous new physicians make premature medication changes that have led to manic rages, violence, suicide attempts, hospitalizations, or other untoward results of decompensation.

I am reminded of the quotation by Robert Shuman in his compelling book, *The Psychology of Chronic Illness*:

> "When the worlds of patients, families, and physicians meet, however, the results can be collaboration, collision, or indifference."[2]

Family concerns about rash treatment decisions made by a new physician are hardly limited to psychiatric medications. Chronic diseases leading to deterioration in functioning and chronic pain are often hotbeds of complex trials and errors with medications in which our patients often feel that they have been "put through the grinder." Illnesses, such as lupus, multiple sclerosis, rheumatoid arthritis, diabetes, kidney failure, CHF, and all chronic pain syndromes, including burn recovery, are often battlefields in which the patient is desperately seeking some combination of medications and treatments that will bring relief. If, after years of trial and error, a regimen has been found that has brought some modicum of relief, both patients and family members may be extremely anxious that a new physician is about "to muck it all up."

Assuming that confidentiality issues have been adequately addressed, the following statements can go a long way toward assuring that initial meetings with the family members of patients coping with serious mental or physical illnesses result in collaboration not collision:

> "You know, Mrs. Jones, one thing I want to reassure you is that I not only value your input, I need it. Sometimes family mem-

bers get worried that a new physician is going to make quick medication changes that cause problems. I just want to let you know that I'm not going to do that. I need to see what you think is working or has worked in the past. After I get a good feel for your son's condition and which meds have worked and why, only then will I consider changes, and I'll want your input about them. How does that sound to you?"

PRESCRIBING NEW MEDICATIONS TO WELL-KNOWN PATIENTS

The following tips are useful with new patients as well as ongoing patients. But in this section we will focus upon those situations in which we are changing medications in a well-known patient to gain better control of a long-term illness or introducing medications for a new illness in such a patient.

INTERVIEWING TIP #34:   Asking for the Patient's Recommendations for a Medication of Choice

At a recent workshop, a physician, Mark Bernstein, provided a simple suggestion that I have found to be surprisingly useful. Bernstein notes that many patients have preconceived ideas about what medications may be of value to them. As we saw in our last chapter, many times these opinions are often based upon input from family members and/or friends, as well as being the result of "direct to consumer" advertising by pharmaceutical houses. Whatever the source, one can quickly foster a collaborative relationship by asking for the patient's opinion about medication options before offering his or her own recommendation as with:

"Do you have a medication in mind that you might want to take?"

The apparent simplicity of this tip betrays a wealth of complexities. This question immediately places the patient's opinion where it ought to be, at the forefront of the prescribing clinician's mind. The patient may have excellent ideas as to which medications may be effective, or the patient may have some misinformation about specific medications that can be easily corrected.

The patient's answer may also, indirectly, open the door to an understanding of influential "committee lobbyists," ranging from family members to Webmasters, who may have been the originators of the patient's interest or disinterest in a particular medication. With the use of this question, the clinician may also become aware of important patient biases, both "for" and "against" a specific medication, that, if left undetected, could be the determining factors as to whether a medication ever leaves the inside of its bottle.

In a similar vein, if patients are not assertive enough to spontaneously suggest medications that they have their "hearts set on getting," they may leave the office disappointed with their prescriptions. Such prescriptions have an uncanny knack of ending up in wastepaper baskets. The previously described tip ensures that such a hidden disappointment cannot occur. We might still not write the prescription the patient requests, if we feel it is inappropriate, but at least we will have been able to discuss our reasoning and, in the process, modeled a method of sharing medication information with the patient.

This tip also raises the value of uncovering a valid, not sugar coated, idea of the patient's initial gut feelings about taking a newly prescribed medication. No reason exists for us to not be privy to this vital information regarding medication interest before the patient leaves our office, because all we have to do is ask. Once again, the very act of asking for the patient's opinion metacommunicates that we value it. Such interviewing techniques continue to underscore our desire to be an ally with the patient against his or her disease not an opponent against his or her opinions.

In a similar vein, I sometimes precede the above question with the even broader question, "What do you think might help with your symptoms?" Such a question allows the patient to suggest alternative methods of healing other than medications, which may, indeed, be excellent first choices for intervention with some problems and for some patients.

INTERVIEWING TIP #35:   Gauging Initial Receptivity to Prescription
                                                                            Recommendations

Sometimes patients, because of their own anxieties, social hesitancies, or feelings of being rushed, don't really "come clean" with their ambivalent feelings about a new medication. If they walk out of our office, and these vague fears have not been addressed, even though they may outwardly have agreed to take the medication, they have often inwardly decided not to. The result may well be a "no-show" at the next appointment or a patient who, indeed, shows up, but shows up without the prescribed medication in his or her bloodstream. The clinician can use any one or more of the following questions (or come up with a new inquiry) to directly uncover such potential ambivalence:

1. "What are your thoughts about starting up on this med?"
2. "Now that I've talked about all of the benefits and potential common side effects, what are your thoughts about whether or not you think this medication is worth a try?"
3. "What's most appealing to you about trying this med?"
4. "What concerns, if any, do you have about trying this med?"

The trick is to get this stuff "out on the table" rapidly, before any final decision is made by the patient. I have been consistently pleased by the openness of patients to share their opinions on these critical matters, if I just take the time to ask.

Moreover, I have sometimes found that the patient's advice is sound, and my initial choice of a medication was not a good one.

I remember an articulate woman who was a bank manager suffering with a depression. She presented with jet-black hair, lips lightly pursed with red lipstick, and a dusting of rouge on her cheeks. Her dress was that of a sharp business woman, a gray three-piece business suit and newly polished shoes, heels neither too high nor too low. Despite her apparent confidence in the business world, she had a deeply imbedded need to please, part of the reason she had appeared for therapy.

True to form, as I described the antidepressant I was recommending, she thoughtfully nodded her head, and seemed politely interested. But when I asked, "What are your thoughts about starting up on this med?" she commented, "I think it sounds like a pretty good idea, but both my mother and sister tried that medication and got horrible nausea from it. They hated it. But I guess I'll try it, if you think it will help."

Although I should have gathered this family information earlier in the interview, for whatever reason it hadn't surfaced. Clearly, this was not the best first choice of an antidepressant for this patient. I never would have heard this information, unless I had asked the question that I did. She knew this was not the right medication for her. Now I did. Technique counts.

INTERVIEWING TIP #36:   Providing a Medication Menu

While giving a workshop in Ohio, Joseph Holtel, a doctor of osteopathy (DO), offered a useful method of nurturing a collaborative relationship when prescribing a new medication. Many illnesses may have various different appropriate medications or alternative methods of beginning therapy, ranging from medication classes that may have many different medication options within them (antihypertensives, antidepressants) to nonmedical interventions for diabetes and heart disease (exercise, diet).

In these instances, Holtel, using antidepressants as an example, suggests that instead of making a medication recommendation, the clinician shares some information about the pros and cons of each of the possible medications, including specific pros (rapidly helps with sleep, particularly good with anxiety) and specific cons (may cause sleep disturbance, may impair sexual dysfunction). The clinician then asks patients which one they think they might like to try.

I find that this approach can be useful for three reasons:

1. It optimizes the patient's ability to wisely select his or her own medication. I find that patients tolerate side effects better if they helped to choose the medication themselves.
2. It metacommunicates that we have many alternative medications available if the selected medication is less than optimal in relieving symptoms.
3. It provides a platform for the patient to describe in his or her own words to lobbyists, such as family members and friends, why a specific medication is being used when their family and friends may have had preconceived ideas of which medication should be used.

INTERVIEWING TIP #37:   Not Pushing the Initial Decision

Occasionally, the first time we raise the possibility of using a medication, the patient is flooded with both new information and ambivalence, and, consequently, it may not be wise to press for commitment at such moments. This can be particularly true of antidepressants when they are used in a primary care setting, where patients are sometimes worried about the stigma of being placed on such drugs. Although the hectic pace of such clinics often pressures us to make rapid interventions, it is often best to not push a patient to make up his or her mind. An ideal medication that a patient does not want to take is not an ideal medication; it is a medication doomed to never leave the confines of the patient's medicine cabinet.

If you have suggested an antidepressant and the patient looks hesitant to begin it, even after you have spent considerable time exploring the patient's concerns, it may be wise to give the patient more time to contemplate the decision. Any pressure in the first meeting may feel oppositional to the patient and is counterindicated in our medication interest model.

Nothing is worse for long-term medication interest than to have a patient half-heartedly agree to start a medication and then, once home, decide it is not such a "hot idea" to start this thing or, if started, to stay on it. Once deciding not to take a medication or to stop taking one, it is very hard to convince a patient to restart, because, if a patient restarts a medication, the patient must first admit that he or she was wrong to stop it in the first place, hardly a fun thing to do. These "restarted" patients are highly prone to once again stop the medication in order to prove the correctness of their initial decision. The following comments can be effective at giving patients the needed time to make a well-informed decision with which they are comfortable:

> "You know, Mike, I can sense you are still a little hesitant to start on this antidepressant. That's fine. It's smart too. You should take time to weigh the pros and cons of any medicine before you try it.
> "In fact, I don't want you to make your decision today. I think it's much smarter to give it some thought, talk it over with your wife or friends if you want to, and next time we'll review the pros and cons again. If you are still having some concerns then, we'll discuss them and see if we think it's a good idea to try the medication or not. Remember, if you don't like how it is working, you can always stop it.
> "I have a good gut feeling you will really like how you feel on it. I have had some excellent luck with this medication with a lot of patients. But there is absolutely no reason to rush into a decision.
> "Here is some more information on it; read it and see what you think. In my opinion it is very important that you person-

ally be comfortable with a medication before you start it. Does that sound like a good plan to you?"

Sometimes, with patients who really enjoy reading, there are specific books that are valuable in helping them make up their minds about trying psychotropic medications. Ron Green, the residency director in psychiatry at the Dartmouth Medical School has told me that he often suggests, to his more hesitant patients, that they not make up their minds about starting an antidepressant until they have read the book, *When Words are Not Enough, the Women's Prescription for Depression and Anxiety* by Valerie Davis Raskin.[3] After reading the book, many of the patients return with a genuine interest in trying medications, buffered by the reassuring fact that they are making up their own minds, not merely demurring to the mind of their doctor.

The bottom line is a simple one. One of the keys to finding out whether patients genuinely want to start a medication is to give them the time to make their own choice at their own pace. If we rush a prescription onto a patient who really has not made up his or her own mind, we are probably writing a prescription for a patient who will not be filling it.

INTERVIEWING TIP #38:   Keeping Tabs on Mom and Dad

As I end this section I am reminded of one of my favorite tips that was provided by a pediatrician, Dipankar Mukhopadhyay, which delightfully captures the magic and unique solutions sometimes required when working with small children. If you have built up a good ongoing relationship with a child and his or her parents, the following approach can be both great fun and highly effective for improving medication interest in a small child.

The tip addresses a common problem in pediatrics: toddlers fussing about taking medications. Sometimes it is hard for small children to truly understand why they are taking medications, and once they decide they don't want to be bothered, tantrums and tightly clamped lips are not far behind.

The tip is based upon the fact that little kids sometimes get a kick out of the idea that they have to "keep tabs" on Mom or Dad rather than vice versa. This phenomenon can be put to good use in helping kids get interested in taking their medications. After writing out the script, the clinician turns and hands the script to the young patient, saying:

> "Now this piece of paper will allow you to get your medicine from the pharmacist. This medicine will really help your sore throat to feel much better. But the only way it will work is if your Mom remembers to give it to you once in the morning and once at bedtime. Do you think you can make sure your Mom remembers to do this?"

Engaging these young patients in the "monitoring" of their parents' behavior usually gets a chuckle from the parent and an enthusiastic nod from the child. This technique is a wonderful example of "externalizing the problematic behavior," a technique often useful in children and adolescents. For instance, a child who has been teasing another child may be told that there are problems with teasing at school (and why it is a problem) and then may be asked to help make sure it is not happening anymore in the hallways, perhaps being used as a hallway monitor. You may be able to find other uses for "externalizing problematic behaviors" when attempting to increase medication interest even with adults.

MEDICATION INTEREST AND FOLLOW-UP MED CHECKS: A SECOND GLANCE

The hallmark of the medication interest model is the consistent detail given to carefully phrasing questions and comments in such a way as to foster a sense of ongoing alliance in contrast to a feeling of opposition. In the first part of this chapter we have seen that our choice of words plays a pivotal role in creating a sense of collaboration from the first minutes of the initial meeting to those moments when we are introducing new medications to well-known patients. We will now wrap up the chapter, by looking at the power of our words to shape the ongoing alliance in our follow-up med checks, as our patients raise their side-effects, fears, hopes, and successes regarding their current medication regimens.

INTERVIEWING TIP #39:   Aligning with the Patient's Frustration

   As our patients struggle with their symptoms and side effects, many become both frustrated and demoralized. They can grow tired of a seemingly endless stream of medications that seem to go nowhere and sometimes seem to create more problems than they solve. Their reaction is both logical and natural. It is frustrating for us as well.

   As we learned in Chapter 7 with "the shame cycle" that was triggered by missed doses, a subtle deterioration can creep into the ongoing alliance at these junctures, if we are not careful. Some patients may feel a gnawing guilt that they have lost motivation to try new medications, and, if they have a particularly strong alliance with us, they may develop more damaging feelings of guilt and shame, as if they are letting us down. Such feelings can generate a withdrawal of the patient from the therapeutic alliance, reflected by occasional "no-shows," less animated sessions, and less open discussion of their frustrations and concerns, because they fear that such expressions may be interpreted by the physician as a lack of motivation or confidence in the physician.

   A child and adolescent psychiatrist at one of my workshops in Waco, Texas, shared a finely worded statement, that immediately allies the physician with the patient's own feelings of frustration; it is a statement that is made to a patient, who has just had a series of medication failures and is now being started up on "yet another drug."

   I have found it to be very useful at circumventing the potentially disengaging process described above, because it lets the patient know that we too are frustrated, and we are not just making a new recommendation for the "hell of it"; we are looking for something that truly helps. See what you think:

> "You know what? What we want with this new medication is not just the same old same old. What we want is something that is better, not just different. We want you to feel better. If we just get different, then we have to take another look at our plan. We will keep working together till we find something that helps and really helps, and I think we will."

INTERVIEWING TIP #40: The Humor of Discontinuance

Here is a technique that can only be used with a patient well known to us, in which we have developed a relaxed and comfortable bond. These are the delightful types of relationships we forge where humor and laughter play a refreshing counterpoint to our trials and tribulations as we jointly battle against the patient's long-term illness. With such patients we often develop a keen sense of intuition for them and they of us.

If after you have discussed a new medication and a patient agrees to take it, but, nonverbally the patient doesn't seem to be jumping up and down with enthusiasm about the medication, just ask, candidly, what he or she intends to do:

> "You know, Mike, I'm getting the feeling that you are just a bit hesitant to start this med. Which is okay, but I just have a hunch here (well-timed pause) you're not going to take this thing, are you?"

Said with gentle wryness, and with absolutely no tone of condemnation, this technique, if the physician's intuition is on the mark, often results in a smile from the patient, not unlike the smile of a kid caught with his hand in the cookie jar. Once the patient's misgivings are out on the table, productive joint treatment planning can resume.

INTERVIEWING TIP #41:   Collaborating on How Much and When

Side effects are problematic and are often dose-related. As a patient weighs the pros and cons, the severity of side effects, at recommended doses, may outweigh the benefits. A patient may simply say, "I can't take this medication at this dose." At such times, it is important to remember, that, during our medical training, we were fed bell curves and statistics that purport to tell us what the "minimum effective dose" for any medication may be, but these parameters are not necessarily true for all patients. Some people, such as slow metabolizers, lie outside our bell curves and may respond to a medication at lower doses than the recommended dose. Such patients are also more likely to suffer problematic dose-related side effects even at the lower end of the recommended dosage range. We don't always know which patient is going to respond in which way to a medication dosage. Sometimes this situation can provide creative openings to try surprisingly low dosing levels with patients suffering from intolerable side effects. If the following can be done safely from a medical standpoint, it offers a way to collaboratively try a lower dose:

"Mrs. Mack, it looks like the dizziness is just not going to go away, and I totally agree that it is a side effect that simply is too problematic to tolerate, despite the fact that we are getting some good control of your blood pressure. I have an idea. Some people can still get good effects from medications at lower doses. I suggest we try your medication at a lower dose than it is usually given, and see if it still helps with your blood pressure while also seeing if the dizziness goes away. It might not work, but we can at least try it and see what happens. I know that you are uncomfortable with the current dose and I can see why. I'm wondering, what dose of this medication might you feel comfortable taking, say for the next week or two to see what happens?"

If the patient's requested dosage is reasonable and safe, a trial can be tried. I find that patients feel comfortable and pleasantly surprised that their own input is so influential and valued by the physician. In some instances, the lower dose proves inadequate, but I have been pleasantly surprised at how often a lower dose provides good relief with an acceptable side-effect profile.

By the way, from a forensic standpoint, if you choose to try a dose lower than recommended, be sure to write in your note exactly why you are doing so. Obviously, if the lower dose proves to be inadequate, you will need to search for another good medication if one is available or try to see whether there are unexplored ways of helping the patient tolerate the side effects at the necessary higher dose.

A similar strategy can be useful when first starting a medication in which the patient appears wary of the dosage or the medication itself. In such instances, the clinician can suggest starting at a very low dose, telling the patient, "Let's start really low. See how you feel after a couple of weeks, and I think you will feel pretty good, at which point you can decide to raise the dose to the normal level. It's up to you; you call the shot. And next time we meet we'll see how things are going at whatever dose you're on and decide our next step to getting you maximum relief." This strategy maximizes the patient's sense of control. I find that patients frequently return having raised the dose to the desired level.

Similarly, sometimes a patient simply cannot remember to take a medication at a certain "ideal time." For instance, a patient taking a medication t.i.d. may consistently miss the midday dose. Once again, although the recommended t.i.d. dose is most effective, one can sometimes try a b.i.d. dosing, with slightly increased dosage at the b.i.d. doses as partial compensation for the missed middle dose. Obviously, the smoothness of blood level will be affected, but the medication regimen may still be effective. Indeed, this b.i.d. dosing, that the patient enthusiastically embraces, is bound to be more effective than the recommended t.i.d. dose that is almost always missed, and which the patient eventually stops altogether, "because Dr. Shea told me it only works if I take it three times a day." Once again, an ideal treatment plan that the patient cannot do is not ideal. It is a failure.

INTERVIEWING TIP #42: Negotiating a Short-Term Contract

When we tell a patient that it will be necessary to be on a medication for life, the news is difficult to digest, especially if the medication has major side effects and long-term risks, such as liver disease or kidney disease. It is only natural for a patient to balk at such a disconcerting picture of the future. The cons of the medication have just skyrocketed.

Linda Cunning, a physician from one of my workshops in Wisconsin, has come up with a psychologically savvy fashion of working with patients on this issue. The trick is to be the first one to acknowledge the difficulties inherent in agreeing to take a medication (such as lithium) indefinitely, with phrasing such as the following:

> "You know, Mr. Johnson, it really isn't reasonable to commit to taking a medication for the rest of your life. I couldn't do it. Life is complicated. Things change. I know that. On the other hand, because this lithium is so valuable for you in helping you control your bipolar disorder, let's try something in much smaller steps, something that is reasonable and practical. Why don't we contract that you will take the lithium for just a year. At the end of that year, we will see how it is helping and then we can contract for another year if you think it is working well for you. One year at a time. Now that length of time is much more manageable for making a contract. What do you think?"

Nice touch. The technique fits the medication interest model perfectly, with the patient and clinician jointly recognizing the difficulties of maintaining medication interest over time. Together, with the patient calling the final shot, a mutually reasonable contract is created.

INTERVIEWING TIP #43: Expressing Interest in Alternative
Treatments

In the initial interview, I make an effort during my medication history to ask about the topic of "alternative medicines," which play a major role in our culture today. Sometimes the patient does not become interested in alternative treatments until long into our relationship. Whether it is in the initial interview or during one of our ongoing sessions, I tend to use the same approach: an open and nonjudgmental interest in what the patient is doing.

The topic of alternative medicine, if not handled properly, can become a major trip wire into an oppositional relationship instead of a partnership. Some patients are so convinced that their physician is going to be opposed to alternative approaches, that the patients simply do not bring them up, even though they are concurrently seeing an herbalist, acupuncturist, or chiropractor. Such a lack of openness and trust does not bode well for a long-term partnership between a physician and a patient.

Fortunately, I seldom encounter a problem here, because I am genuinely open to new ideas and feel quite certain that techniques, such as acupuncture, can be efficacious. This unexpected openness, once again, assures the patient that we are not opponents – we are trusted allies.

If a patient comments that he or she is trying an herbal remedy or some other alternative practice, I always ask, "Oh, do you think it is helping?" If they say it is, I enthusiastically comment, "then by all means you should keep using it." Patients are genuinely pleased by this unanticipated response on my part. I then proceed to share the following:

"Some people think that all physicians are highly opposed to alternative medicine. This is simply not true. I feel certain there are many things that we will learn about healing from many different systems. Indeed, digitalis, a great heart medication, was first used as an herbal remedy centuries ago. I myself have found that acupuncture can be helpful in certain pain conditions.

"My only cautionary note is that, in some instances, only a standard medication will, in my opinion, provide the necessary relief or cure. In these instances, it is critical not to stop the medication. I will always give you my best medical advice on whether you should try a specific alternative technique. That's my job as your physician. Also, always let me know if you are thinking of starting on any vitamin or herb or supplement, because these agents can interact with medications, sometimes causing unwanted side effects.

"I am also very eager to talk with your alternative specialist to share what I am doing and how it is helping, and to hear the same about their approaches. There are several alternative specialists in the area with whom I have a good working relationship.

"One final thing. As you can see from my openness to alternative methods, I believe that good healers have a keen interest in what other healers are doing. If you bump into an alternative specialist that in any way begins to knock my medications or what I am doing, beware of them. They clearly are not open healers. Their bad-mouthing of my methods should alert you to go elsewhere, so that we can find someone who wants to join our team not someone who wants to destroy it, because we got a great team going here."

I have never had this approach backfire. On the other hand, I have had some patients switch alternative healers because they did not like the healer's attitudes toward me. As we can see, this nonoppositional approach, that fosters an ongoing collaborative feeling, has transformed a potentially oppositional trap into an opportunity for an even stronger alliance.

Medication Interest: Final Reflections

As physicians, and all other clinicians who prescribe medications, it is our mission to help patients find relief from, and sometimes even cure of, the many illnesses that plague them. The task is difficult, and we certainly do not pretend that we can always succeed to the degree that we wish. Undoubtedly, our medications play a major role in the healing process. But it is our relationships with our patients that determine whether these medications will even get their chance to heal.

Whether we are a primary care physician helping a patient with the ravages of AIDS or a psychiatrist helping a patient to overcome the horrors of schizophrenia, it is ultimately our relationship that heals not our medications, because it is our relationships that get the medications out of their bottles.

Medicine always was and always will be an art. Whether they meet us in the hectic halls of a primary care clinic or the frenetic waiting rooms of a packed community mental health center, there will always be patients, who are deeply frightened and in great pain. These patients will never forget the physicians who listened to their hopes and concerns about their medications with a sense of compassion and talked with them about the pros and cons of their medications with skill.

As Francis Peabody said, "the secret of the care of the patient is in caring for the patient." We might only add that caring is always good, but caring with skill is even better. It is to a deepening of Peabody's sense of caring and to the development of those interviewing skills that can enhance that caring, that we have dedicated ourselves in the pages of this book.

REFERENCES

1. Peabody F. A medical classic: the care of the patient by Francis W. Peabody. *JAMA* 1927;88:877.
2. Shuman R. *The Psychology of Chronic Illness: the Healing Work of Patients, Therapists, & Families.* New York: Basic Books, 1996:84.
3. Raskin VD. *When Words are Not Enough, the Women's Prescription for Depression and Anxiety.* New York: Broadway Books, 1997.

Tip Archive: "Quick Reference"

To the reader: For fast recall/reference, all interviewing tips are listed here in their order of appearance and by name. The wording of the tips is exactly as it appears in the text, and the reader is referred to the appropriate page for a more detailed review as desired.

INTERVIEWING TIP #1:   Inquiry into Lost Dreams *(see page 28)*

"Is there anything that your asthma (use patient's specific disorder) is keeping you from doing that you really wish you could do again?"

Follow-Up 1: "Now I can't promise this, but I have had some very good luck with helping other students, with asthma like yours, to get back into sports. We have some great meds, that can help with that goal. Once again, no promises, but I would like to work with you to see if we might be able to get you back out on that soccer field. How does that sound to you?"

Follow-Up 2: "I know you are getting some tough side effects – and they are tough – but, fortunately, I have some ideas on how we might be able to make them much better, and I don't think we have yet seen the full power of these meds to help you feel better. We are still trying to get you back on that soccer field that we talked about in our first meeting. If you can give me another two weeks to see if I can lower the side effects and get you some better relief from these attacks, I think I might be able to do that. Is it a deal?"

INTERVIEWING TIP #2:   Tapping Family Motivators *(see page 30)*

"Mr. Perez, I know you don't feel much like taking these medications for your diabetes, and I understand that. There might be another reason, in addition to taking care of yourself, why it may be very important for you to try to take them. I think they can help you to take care of your family. You see, your dad's diabetes is what led to his dying from a heart attack at such a young age. These medications can help to make sure that you don't get a heart attack, something that you know from your own experience would be horrible for your wife and kids. We need to keep you healthy, for them. I know it's a nuisance to have to take medications, I really do. I sure don't enjoy taking medications myself, but if it can save your family from that kind of pain, I think it is worth it. What do you think?"

INTERVIEWING TIP #3:   Providing a Visual Reminder for Family
Motivation *(see page 31)*

"Mr. James, we've already decided that one of your reasons, besides taking care of yourself, that you want to stay on your medications for your high blood pressure is to keep healthy for your wife. That's a great goal, and I think you can do it. Some of my patients with a similar goal have found a neat trick to remind them why they are taking their medications. You simply set your pill bottle on a large picture of your family, so that every time you reach for it, you are reminded of what the losses may be to your family if you got a heart attack because of your high blood pressure. Many of my patients say it really helps them to stay motivated. How does that idea sound to you?"

INTERVIEWING TIP #4:   Introducing Medication Interest *(see page 37)*

"My goal as a physician is to always give you my best advice, whether that advice is to start a medication, stay on it, or get off it. Together we want to find a medicine that you are genuinely *interested* in taking because it makes you feel better. You're the one who is putting the medication in your body so it's your opinion that is most important, not mine. So please always let me know exactly what you think about the meds we are trying. I'm counting on your input. You know your body better than I do. And I think we can be a great team in finding a medication that works well for you – that really makes you feel better. How does that sound to you?"

INTERVIEWING TIP #5:   Exploring Med Sensitivity *(see page 40)*

"Do you think that you are particularly sensitive to medications?"

Follow-Up 1: "What are some of the things that you have seen in the past with medications that has shown you that you are oversensitive?"

Follow-Up 2: Do not challenge the patient's self-perception of being "oversensitive" even if it is inaccurate.

Follow-Up 3: "Would it be okay with you, if I start you off at one-half of the recommended starting dose for this medication, because of your concerns about being sensitive to meds? I think this would be a smart way to start you off. I call this a *baby dose* of the med, and I think it is a very gentle way to begin medications. This way, your body can get a feel for the med first before we give you much of a dose. Any side effects, and there might not be any with this little dose, will probably be much smaller in nature. Then when you are feeling comfortable on the medication, we can slowly increase it to get you feeling better and better. I just think this is a smart way for us to start. What do you think?"

INTERVIEWING TIP #6:   The Trap Door Question: Ascertaining
the Patient's View of the Current
Dosage *(see page 55)*

"At this point in time, in your own opinion, do you feel that you are on too little, too much, or just the right amount of this medication?"

INTERVIEWING TIP #7:   Family Inquiry on Dosage *(see page 57)*

"How does your spouse (partner) feel about this dosage?"

INTERVIEWING TIP #8:   Introducing Physician Interest in
Hearing About the Pros
and Cons *(see page 61)*

"I have tremendous respect for medications and have found them to be extremely useful in helping my patients. I just want you to know that I also realize that medications can have tough side effects, and I take those side effects very seriously.
"Personally, I only take medications when I feel that I genuinely need them, and I feel that the benefits outweigh the costs. I take the same approach with my patients. So I won't suggest

a medication unless I really have a feeling it will help you. I would never recommend a medication that I myself would not take or give to a member of my own family.
"And I always try to fill in my patients on possible side effects and the pros and cons of using the medication. You are currently on some excellent medicines, and there are some other excellent medicines out there. Our goal is to find the right combination that works best for you. How's that sound?"

Follow-Up: "By the way, if we run into any problems with side effects that lead us to think that the medication is causing more harm than good, I'll be the first one to tell you to get off of it. I'm not here to make you stay on any medication that isn't making you feel better or helping to control your illness in the long run.
"Our goal is to help you find a set of medications that you are genuinely interested in taking because they make you feel better, not because I tell you to take them. I'm always interested in your input, and I have a feeling we might be able to further help your asthma (refer to patient's specific illness). . . . But fill me in for a moment. What has been your impression, overall, on how well your current medications are working out for you?"

INTERVIEWING TIP #9:   Instilling Positive Expectations *(see page 63)*

"This medication has really proven itself in recent research, and I, personally, have had some great luck with it. I would say that in the last two months alone, I've had at least a dozen patients, sitting in that exact chair, who have had very significant improvements in their breathing and ability to get around since we started them on it. There are no guarantees, but it can be really pretty striking how much better people feel when taking it."

INTERVIEWING TIP #10:   The Talisman Effect: Optimizing the
                          Power of the Prescription to
                          Symbolize Hope *(see page 64)*

"Well, good luck with this. I've got a really good feeling it is going to help you."

INTERVIEWING TIP #11:   Ascertaining the Patient's Ongoing
                          Views on Efficacy *(see page 65)*

1. "How's that medication working out for you that we started up last time?"
2. "Is the medication helping with any of your symptoms?"
3. "Are you getting any of the side effects that we mentioned last time?"
4. "Are you having any problems that you are wondering whether or not they may be a side effect?"
5. "What do you think about the medication, so far?"
6. "Do you like the medication, so far?"
7. "Do you feel that the relief you are getting outweighs the side effects you are having at this point in time?"
8. "At this point in time, do you feel that the pros are outweighing the cons with this medication?"

INTERVIEWING TIP #12:   Techniques for Conveying Concern
                          About Side Effects *(see page 67)*

1. "Tell me about a specific time you felt dizzy and walk me through what happened."
2. "Just how bad does the dizziness get?"
3. "How often are you feeling it?"
4. "How many days this week did you get it?"
5. "Is it making it harder for you to do anything?"
6. "On a scale from 1 to 10, with 1 meaning 'it hardly bothers me' and 10 meaning 'I can't stand this side

effect,' where would you put your dizziness this past week?"

7. "I have some ideas about what to do to get rid of the dizziness, but if we can't, do you think the dizziness is bad enough that it outweighs the good things your medication is doing, like making it easier for you to breath and getting rid of some of that swelling in your legs? Sometimes it's a tough call, but only you can make it. The bottom line is do you think you feel better on or off the medication at this point?"

INTERVIEWING TIP #13:   Probing for Impending Discontinuance
(see page 68)

"We've been trying to decrease this side effect, but I know it is still a problem. What kind of thoughts, even fleeting in nature, have you had about maybe stopping the medication?"

INTERVIEWING TIP #14:   Proactively Recommending Discontinuance (see page 69)

"Jim, I just don't like the problem we are having with this side-effect. If we can't get it under control, I really think we may need to stop this med, even though I know it's also helping too. I'm just worried that the pros of using it are being outweighed by the cons. What do you think?"

INTERVIEWING TIP #15:   Gently Exploring Cost Issues (see page 73)

"Mrs. Jackson, I'm always curious on how much my patient's medications cost. How much did you end up having to pay for the (insert medication in question) this past month?"

Follow-Up 1: "Were you surprised by the cost?"

Follow-Up 2: "How much of that did you have to pay for your-self?"

Follow-Up 3: "It can be tough for anyone to pay for their medi-cations; how much of a burden do you think this will be for you and your family?"

INTERVIEWING TIP #16:   Calling in Prescriptions for the Patient
(see page 76)

"Would you like me to call that prescription in for you? Once I've called it in, you won't have to wait as long at the pharmacist and, if you like, someone else could pick up the medication for you. You can even call ahead and make sure the prescription is waiting for you."

INTERVIEWING TIP #17:   Short-Circuiting the Shame Cycle
(see page 79)

"It is very easy to forget to take a dose. If you notice yourself doing that, please note whether there is anything incon-venient about the timing of the dose. You can even make a list if that helps you to remember. But this way, if there are any missed doses, we can put our heads together to see whether we can figure out a better time or an easier way to remember. The bottom line is that I really think this medi-cation can help you, but I want to find a way that is easiest for you to remember to take it. Can you promise to let me know about any missed doses? And we'll see what we can come up with to help. Is that something that you think you can do? It will help us both."

INTERVIEWING TIP #18:   Normalizing Missed Doses (see page 81)

"Mr. Jeffers, many patients tell me that it can be easy to forget to take medications at times (normalization). In the weeks since we last met, how many doses do you think you might have missed per week, just roughly" (gentle assumption).

INTERVIEWING TIP #19:   Exploring Workplace Stigmatization
(see page 82)

"Are you having any problems with taking the pills at work?"

INTERVIEWING TIP #20:   Minimizing Workplace Stigmatization
with the "Vitamin Bottle Decoy" *(see page 82)*

"I have found that there is a very simple way to deal with this
    problem. At home keep your medication in its standard
    bottle. But bring a couple of your pills to work in a tiny, but
    well-labeled empty 'vitamin bottle.' Then you can pull the
    bottle out anytime at lunch or where most appropriate, and,
    if anybody asks, just rave about how much benefit you've
    been getting from vitamin C or whatever vitamin you
    choose to rave about. No one will give it a second thought."

INTERVIEWING TIP #21:   Changing "Tapes" *(see page 89)*

"Take that!"

"Not today you don't."

"This one is for you OCD, I'm gonna kick your butt today."

INTERVIEWING TIP #22:   Dismantling the "Addiction Myth"
(see page 93)

"There is a common misconception about antidepressants, that
    I just wanted to address with you, because you may run
    into it. Many people quite naturally, and you might have
    some of these concerns yourself, are worried that these

medications are addictive. First of all, I would always tell you if a medication I was giving you was addictive or not. Second, these medications simply are not.

"They do not make you high. I have never seen anyone in my entire career crave them; in fact, drug addicts get mad at me if I prescribe them, because they want addictive drugs instead.

"Let me explain exactly how they work. All of our brain cells depend upon small molecules that function as messengers from one cell to the next. These messenger molecules are called *neurotransmitters*. We will simply call them *messengers*.

"With depression you may have low amounts of the messengers called *serotonin* or *norepinephrine*. It is exactly like diabetes, where the patient's pancreas is low on making insulin. The appropriate cure for diabetes is to give the patient insulin so it gets back to a normal level. Insulin is not an addictive medication. We are simply getting the person's insulin level back to normal.

"In depression the brain may be low on serotonin, and so we give the patient a medication that raises the serotonin level back to normal. Serotonin is not addictive, no more than insulin is. Both insulin and serotonin are naturally in your body but low in diabetes and depression."

(I then continue with education on how the medications work, and I may make drawings of the synapse for patients or refer to premade patient educational aids that they can take home.)

Follow-Up 1: "By the way, you may have heard that if you suddenly stop some antidepressants you can get some unwanted side effects, sometimes called the *withdrawal syndrome*. This is because your body has made some small adjustments to the medication over the long term. It is not the same as being addicted to a drug. There is no psychological craving for these meds. Moreover, the withdrawal syndrome does not happen if you taper off the medication slowly, which we always would, and I myself have seldom seen problems with this process. Let me explain what symptoms you might get if you suddenly stopped the medication."

(I then proceed to alert the patient to the possible problems that could be encountered.)

INTERVIEWING TIP #23:   Dismantling "the Crutch Myth" *(see page 95)*

"There is another common misconception that these medications are crutches, that somehow you should be able to cope with depression without medications. But if your brain is not making enough serotonin, it simply isn't making enough serotonin, and you can't just 'will it' to make more, any more than a person with diabetes can will their pancreas to make more insulin. We would never tell a person with diabetes that their insulin is a crutch because it isn't. We are simply getting their insulin back to the normal level that everyone else has.

"It is exactly the same with your depression. Your brain is not making enough serotonin, and we are just going to get your serotonin back to the normal level that everybody else has. It isn't a crutch. It is getting your serotonin level back to normal, so that you then have a fair chance to effectively cope with your stresses. Don't let anyone tell you it is a crutch, because it is simply not true."

INTERVIEWING TIP #24:   Getting a Read on the Patient's
                          Medication Grapevine *(see page 96)*

"Sometimes this medication can help with problems like you are having. Have you heard anything good or bad – from the Internet, magazines, radio, or television – about this medication?"

INTERVIEWING TIP #25:   Testing the Waters *(see page 99)*

"Jim, you've been doing great on your medications now for over a year. It's wonderful that you have your bipolar disorder (substitute whatever illness the patient is dealing with) in excellent control. Some of my patients tell me that after awhile, they get curious about whether or not they still have the bipolar disorder or even need the medications. I think that is a natural curiosity. Do you ever have thoughts like that?"

INTERVIEWING TIP #26:   Probing for Resistance from the Patient's Spouse/Partner *(see page 102)*

"How do you think your spouse (partner) will feel about your starting on an antidepressant?"

INTERVIEWING TIP #27:   Anticipating Friends' Opinions on Medications *(see page 103)*

1. "Do you have any friends who have taken this medication, and, if so, what did they think of it?"
2. "Have you heard anything good or bad about this medication from other patients (consumers/clients)?"

INTERVIEWING TIP #28:   Looking for Bad Associations That a Teenager May Have with a Medication *(see page 104)*

"Do you have any friends or know of anyone at school who has taken this medication?"

INTERVIEWING TIP #29:   Selective Use of Clinician
"Self-Transparency" *(see page 105)*

1. "You know, my mother is on this medication and thinks it is just great."
2. "You know, Jim, I've been on this same medication for my high blood pressure for years, and it has been a super med for me. My blood pressure has been great and any side effects went away quickly."

INTERVIEWING TIP #30:   Finding the Patient's Personal Target
Symptoms *(see page 113)*

1. "Mrs. Davis, of all of the different symptoms that you are getting from your heart problems, what are the ones that are most problematic for you?"
2. "Mrs. Davis, of all of your different heart symptoms, which are the ones you most want help with?"
3. "Mrs. Davis, if I had a magic pill, and I don't, but if I did, and it could completely take away just one of your symptoms, which one would you want me to get rid of?"

INTERVIEWING TIP #31:   Eliciting the Patient's Views on Current
Medications *(see page 114)*

1. "What is your understanding of the purpose of each of your medications?"
2. "Do they seem to help?"
3. "Do some help better than others?"
4. "Do you like your medications?"
5. "Were you interested in making any changes in any of them?"
6. "Do you think that you need to be on medications?"
7. "Have you ever thought of alternative treatments in addition to your medications or perhaps instead of them?"

INTERVIEWING TIP #32:   Eliciting Children's Views on Their
Medications *(see page 115)*

1. "Why do you think you are taking this pill?"
2. "How is it supposed to help you?"
3. "Do you want to be taking it?"

INTERVIEWING TIP #33:   Reassuring Family Members that No
Hasty Decisions are About
to Be Made *(see page 116)*

"You know, Mrs. Jones, one thing I want to reassure you is
that I not only value your input, I need it. Sometimes family members get worried that a new physician is going to
make quick medication changes that cause problems. I just
want to let you know that I'm not going to do that. I need
to see what you think is working or has worked in the past.
After I get a good feel for your son's condition and which
meds have worked and why, only then will I consider
changes, and I'll want your input about them. How does
that sound to you?"

INTERVIEWING TIP #34:   Asking for the Patient's
Recommendations for a
Medication of Choice *(see page 118)*

"Do you have a medication in mind that you might want to
take?"

INTERVIEWING TIP #35:   Gauging Initial Receptivity to
Prescription Recommendations *(see page 120)*

1. "What are your thoughts about starting up on this med?"
2. "Now that I've talked about all of the benefits and potential
common side effects, what are your thoughts about whether or not you think this medication is worth a try?"

3. "What's most appealing to you about trying this med?"
4. "What concerns, if any, do you have about trying this med?"

INTERVIEWING TIP #36:   Providing a Medication Menu *(see page 121)*

When helping a patient choose a medication, in this technique the clinician refrains from making a specific suggestion. Instead – using antidepressants as an example – the clinician shares some information about the pros and cons of each of the possible medications, including specific pros (rapidly helps with sleep, particularly good with anxiety) and specific cons (may cause sleep disturbance, may impair sexual dysfunction). The clinician then asks patients which one they think they might like to try.

INTERVIEWING TIP #37:   Not Pushing the Initial Decision
(see page 122)

"You know, Mike, I can sense you are still a little hesitant to start on this antidepressant. That's fine. It's smart too. You should take time to weigh the pros and cons of any medicine before you try it.
"In fact, I don't want you to make your decision today. I think it's much smarter to give it some thought, talk it over with your wife or friends if you want to, and next time we'll review the pros and cons again. If you are still having some concerns then, we'll discuss them and see if we think it's a good idea to try the medication or not. Remember, if you don't like how it is working, you can always stop it.
"I have a good gut feeling you will really like how you feel on it. I have had some excellent luck with this medication with a lot of patients. But there is absolutely no reason to rush into a decision.
"Here is some more information on it; read it and see what you think. In my opinion, it is very important that you per-

sonally be comfortable with a medication before you start
it. Does that sound like a good plan to you?"

INTERVIEWING TIP #38:   Keeping Tabs on Mom and Dad
(see page 124)

"Now this piece of paper will allow you to get your medicine
from the pharmacist. This medicine will really help your
sore throat to feel much better. But the only way it will
work is if your Mom remembers to give it to you once in
the morning and once at bedtime. Do you think you can
make sure your Mom remembers to do this?"

INTERVIEWING TIP #39:   Aligning with the Patient's Frustration
(see page 126)

"You know what? What we want with this new medication is
not just the same old same old. What we want is something
that is better, not just different. We want you to feel better.
If we just get different, then we have to take another look
at our plan. We will keep working together till we find
something that helps, and I think we will."

INTERVIEWING TIP #40:   The Humor of Discontinuance *(see page 127)*

"You know, Mike, I'm getting the feeling that you are just a bit
hesitant to start this med. Which is okay, but I just have a
hunch here (well-timed pause) you're not going to take this
thing, are you?"

INTERVIEWING TIP #41:   Collaborating on How Much and
When *(see page 128)*

"Mrs. Mack, it looks like the dizziness is just not going to go
away, and I totally agree that it is a side effect that simply is too problematic to tolerate, despite the fact that we

are getting some good control of your blood pressure. I have an idea. Some people can still get good effects from medications at lower doses. I suggest we try your medication at a lower dose than it is usually given and see if it still helps with your blood pressure while also seeing if the dizziness goes away. It might not work, but we can at least try it and see what happens. I know that you are uncomfortable with the current dose and I can see why. I'm wondering, what dose of this medication might you feel comfortable taking, say for the next week or two to see what happens?"

Alternative when First Starting a Med: "Let's start really low. See how you feel after a couple of weeks, and I think you will feel pretty good, at which point you can decide to raise the dose to the normal level. It's up to you; you call the shot. And next time we meet we'll see how things are going at whatever dose you're on and decide our next step to getting you maximum relief."

INTERVIEWING TIP #42: Negotiating a Short-Term Contract
(see page 130)

"You know, Mr. Johnson, it really isn't reasonable to commit to taking a medication for the rest of your life. I couldn't do it. Life is complicated. Things change. I know that. On the other hand, because this lithium is so valuable for you in helping you control your bipolar disorder, let's try something in much smaller steps, something that is reasonable and practical. Why don't we contract that you will take the lithium for just a year. At the end of that year, we will see how it is helping and then we can contract for another year if you think it is working well for you. One year at a time. Now that length of time is much more manageable for making a contract. What do you think?"

INTERVIEWING TIP #43:   Expressing Interest in Alternative
Treatments *(see page 130)*

"Some people think that all physicians are highly opposed to
alternative medicine. That is simply not true. I feel certain
there are many things that we will learn about healing
from many different systems. Indeed, digitalis, a great
heart medication, was first used as an herbal remedy centuries ago. I myself have found that acupuncture can be
helpful in certain pain conditions.

"My only cautionary note is that, in some instances, only a
standard medication will, in my opinion, provide the necessary relief or cure. In these instances, it is critical not to
stop the medication. I will always give you my best medical advice on whether you should try a specific alternative
technique. That's my job as your physician. Also, always
let me know if you are thinking of starting on any vitamin
or herb or supplement, because these agents can interact with medications, sometimes causing unwanted side
effects.

"I am also very eager to talk with your alternative specialist to
share what I am doing and how it is helping, and to hear
the same about their approaches. There are several alternative specialists in the area with whom I have a good working relationship.

"One final thing. As you can see from my openness to alternative methods, I believe that good healers have a keen
interest in what other healers are doing. If you bump into
an alternative specialist that in any way begins to knock
my medications or what I am doing, beware of them. They
clearly are not open healers. Their bad-mouthing of my
methods should alert you to go elsewhere, so that we can
find someone who wants to join our team not someone
who wants to destroy it, because we got a great team going
here."

INDEX